THE
ketogenic
DIET

The Scientifically Proven Approach to Fast, Healthy Weight Loss

KRISTEN MANCINELLI, MS, RD

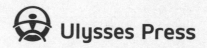 Ulysses Press

Published by
Ulysses Press
P.O. Box 3440
Berkeley, CA 94703
www.ulyssespress.com

ISBN: 978-1-61243-394-3
Library of Congress Catalog Number 2014943031

Printed in Canada by Marquis Book Printing

20 19 18 17 16 15 14 13 12 11 10 9

Acquisitions Editor: Katherine Furman
Managing Editor: Claire Chun
Editor: Renee Rutledge
Proofreader: Lauren Harrison
Indexer: Sayre Van Young
Cover design: Double R Design
Interior design: what!design @ whatweb.com
Layout: Jake Flaherty

Distributed by Publishers Group West

IMPORTANT NOTE TO READERS
This book has been written and published strictly for informational and educational purposes only. It is not intended to serve as medical advice or to be any form of medical treatment. You should always consult your physician before altering or changing any aspect of your medical treatment and/or undertaking a diet regimen, including the guidelines as described in this book. Do not stop or change any prescription medications without the guidance and advice of your physician. Any use of the information in this book is made on the reader's good judgment after consulting with his or her physician and is the reader's sole responsibility. This book is not intended to diagnose or treat any medical condition and is not a substitute for a physician.

This book is independently authored and published and no sponsorship or endorsement of this book by, and no affiliation with, any trademarked brands or other products mentioned within is claimed or suggested. All trademarks that appear in this book belong to their respective owners and are used here for informational purposes only. The author and publishers encourage readers to patronize the quality brands and products mentioned in this book.

To my teachers, Joan and Toni, who taught me to read thoroughly, observe carefully, and draw my own conclusions—even if we disagree. To Cedar and Higgins, my LA family. And finally to Mark, Michelle, Duncan, Brian, Austin, Aaron, and everyone at "the office."

Contents

Foreword

Conventional wisdom says that if you want to lose weight and get healthy you need to cut down on the amount of fat you consume, control the portion sizes of your food to lower your calorie intake, eats lots of healthy whole grains as well as unlimited fruits and vegetables, and exercise on the treadmill for at least an hour a day. Anytime you want to get serious about your diet and lifestyle, these beliefs automatically become the default. But have you ever stopped to ask yourself why you view them as truths? And when these strategies ultimately fail, do you blame yourself for not having enough willpower to make it work? These are just some of the questions that registered dietitian Kristen Mancinelli challenges you to think about in her book.

My name is Jimmy Moore and I am the author of the best-selling 2014 book *Keto Clarity: Your Definitive Guide to the Benefits of a Low-Carb, High-Fat Diet*. I've spent many years researching and personally experimenting with a low-carb, moderate-protein, high-fat diet (aka the ketogenic diet) to examine all the benefits that come from shifting your body from being a sugar-burner to a fat-burner. It's an exciting prospect to think that there is a better alternative to the low-fat, high-carb diets that have dominated people's dietary preferences. I used to be one of those people who believed a low-fat diet was the way to go and my weight and health suffered. By the age of 32, I had gotten all the way up to 410 lbs, wore 62-inch pants and 5XL shirts, and took three prescription medications before I finally came across the information that you will see in the coming pages. Needless to say, it changed my life forever and I'm still (as I like to call it!) livin' la vida low-carb!

The interest in using fat and ketones instead of glucose and carbohydrates as the primary fuel source has grown exponentially in the past few years as mounting research shows that the body and brain actually prefer ketone bodies instead of glucose as the energy source of choice. The problem is the vast majority of people have not been exposed to relevant information clearly explained in convincing, everyday language they can learn from and embrace. Until now.

Mancinelli attempts to lift the stigma associated with the ketogenic diet, though medical practitioners are scared to say the "k" word out of fear of the backlash from patients and colleagues still rooted in the supposed infallibility of more conventional ideas. The fact is our bodies are being flooded with way too many carbohydrates that are raising our blood sugar and insulin levels and increasing the level of inflammation in the body. Inflammation is the true culprit in so many chronic health issues we are dealing with today and yet the focus remains on controlling calories and fat. Does anyone else see what's wrong with this picture? If carbohydrates are contributing to an unhealthy increase in inflammation, blood sugar, and insulin levels, isn't it logical to reduce their consumption in our diets? Of course it is. A bit of common sense should kick in at some point in this discussion.

I'm going to warn you right now that much of the information you will read in this book will challenge you to the very core of what you believe and why you believe it in terms of diet and health. But I urge you to keep an open mind, absorb what Mancinelli is sharing, consider the arguments and points she makes with a fresh look, and then adjust your thinking accordingly. You will very likely experience a paradigm shift in your thinking that you will then share with friends, coworkers, and family members who need to hear a voice of truth that could very well change their lives forever.

Obesity and chronic disease are not an inevitable fate if you are armed with the information you need to make the best choices for living an optimally healthy life. This book provides you that information. It's up to you to decide whether to continue accepting the conventional wisdom you've embraced for your entire life or consider an alternative point of view that is backed by solid science. I wish you well in your pursuit of a thriving, healthy life.

Jimmy Moore, author of *Keto Clarity*
and owner of "Livin' La Vida Low-Carb"
livinlavidalowcarb.com

Author's Note

I grew up during the low-fat diet craze in the 1980s and '90s. I remember as a child hearing about people on the Atkins diet eating a lot of fat and almost no carbs, and I worried for them. Like most people, I thought fat made you fat—and gave you heart disease to boot. I held on to that conviction in graduate school, where I studied the science of nutrition and public health. Understanding how the body uses fats and carbohydrates, and the role of insulin, gave me a sense that carbs (in the form of sugar and starch) were a much bigger problem than we'd been making them out to be. I remember raising the point once or twice in class: Why did our common nutritional advice not match what we knew about how cells—and ultimately *people*—become fat?

When I finished school and left behind the rigor of the science classroom it was easy to bury my suspicion of "the trouble with carbohydrates" under my sweet tooth and the consensus opinion that there was no such "trouble," after all. But by the time the offer came to write this book, I was well into my career as a dietitian—actually helping people lose weight rather than just theorizing about it. I'd seen many overweight individuals return to a normal size and regain control of their health by sharply reducing carbohydrates. They'd quit eating toast and jam for breakfast and switched to eggs and avocados, making similar changes for meals throughout the day. Within a few weeks, their smiles would grow bigger and their bellies smaller, and they would move into a lower-risk category for heart disease and diabetes. They'd say their doctors told them to eat a low-fat diet, but didn't talk that much about carbs. This is still standard advice for weight loss and overall health. A high-fat, low-carb diet has not, until recently, had very many champions. I myself might not be so bold in advocating for it if I didn't see the results in my daily work with overweight, frustrated individuals for whom carbohydrate restriction offers the first real hope of success.

This book is aimed at overweight adults in otherwise good health. It is not for anyone with a diagnosed (or suspected) health problem, anyone taking medication, children, pregnant women, or the elderly. If you fall into one of these categories you would be wise to consult a registered dietitian or other healthcare provider to guide you in appropriate methods of weight loss. Even if you are in good health, a book is no substitute for individualized attention from a qualified professional, and you may want to consider seeking this type of support to help you achieve your weight-loss goals.

The ketogenic diet is not without its downsides. There are potential side effects; some are relatively benign, like initial fatigue and constipation, and some quite serious, like dehydration or acidosis—which, particularly in diabetics, can be life threatening. People with diabetes, kidney disease, or other metabolic disorders should not attempt ketogenic dieting except under direct medical supervision.

That said, the majority of people with healthy, functioning metabolisms experience rapid weight loss on the ketogenic diet, and, after an initial week or two of unpleasant symptoms, side effects diminish or disappear completely. Energy levels improve, hunger subsides, and the prospect of achieving a normal weight in this lifetime makes the thought of eating a candy bar wholly unappealing.

In the course of my research for this book I spent four months on the ketogenic diet. You can read about my experience in the Introduction to follow. I also spoke to dozens of individuals who practice very-low-carb dieting and/or work with those who do, some of whom are interviewed throughout this book. The field of nutrition science is vast, and constantly expanding; this book is an entry point into the ketogenic diet world, and you will find many resources for further learning in Chapter 13.

Finally, it is not my intention to villainize carbohydrates. Many peoples worldwide live on diets rich in grains and starchy vegetables while maintaining a normal weight. It is true that there is not one "right" diet for everyone, and the ketogenic diet is not the be-all, end-all solution to weight loss. But science and history show that it works, and it is my hope that if you are overweight and want to try very-low-carb dieting, this book will give you the tools to succeed.

My Experience on the Ketogenic Diet

Do you have a fear of fat? I had a fear of carbs.

When I was in graduate school I went through a phase where I more or less refused to eat carbohydrates. I was taking a course on the metabolism of macronutrients that explained what happens on a cellular level when you ingest carbs, fats, and proteins. It was impossible to ignore that the situation I read about in my course texts—the one in which eating carbohydrates caused secretion of insulin, accumulation of fat, and sometime thereafter (depending on how young and fit you were) diabetes—was happening *in my own body.*

Truth be told, I became somewhat terrified of having too much insulin in my blood: terrified that my cells would become resistant to it and I would get diabetes, terrified that the fat would not be able to get out of my fat cells (insulin blocks their exit) and thus I would grow fatter every year of my life as I continued to eat yummy carbohydrates that would jack up my blood sugar and my insulin, and then, when the two would fall, cause me to get another craving for sugary foods that I would ultimately indulge because, well, I was still skinny. But I could see the overweight, diabetic me up ahead, and it wasn't a pretty sight.

So I cut way back on carbs—no muffins, cakes, cookies, or ice cream, and I had only the rare slice of homemade or bakery-fresh bread. I skipped rice or pasta whenever offered, and I simply quit seeking out starches and sugars. I decided to keep apples, more for practicality than anything else: I was a full-time student with two part-time jobs, and apples were easy to throw in my bag for a snack between classes and work. My diet centered on high-quality proteins, non-starchy vegetables, and what were considered "good" fats: the mono and polyunsaturated kind found in most plants and fish. For breakfast I had plain, full-fat yogurt, or a blend I made myself from the plain and the vanilla varieties to make a just-sweet-enough bowl, along with nuts and half an apple cut into pieces. For lunch I had salads or a load of fresh vegetables with a protein item, and for dinner I usually cooked tofu, fish, or lentils with more vegetables. I probably averaged 150 g of carbs per day—not even close to ketogenic. But I sure had the mentality that (starch + sugar) = (fat + diabetes), and I wanted no part of it. On the weekends out to brunch I had an egg omelet with a side salad, hold the potatoes, and thought, "*No way am I eating that toast—do you know what the body does with all that starch?*"

Mind you, I was not overweight, nor close to it: I weighed a perfectly normal 125 lbs for my 5'5" frame. I was active, biking most days to school or work, and working out at the gym a couple of days a week. Yet in the course of this low-carb experiment—which lasted two-and-a-half months—I lost 12 lbs. Being at the time a twenty-something-year-old woman surrounded by media images of unattainable thinness, I wasn't too mad about my new ultrathin frame. I just bought skinnier jeans. My friends gave half compliments touched with concern: "You've lost so much weight! You were so thin already... But you look great!" It was hard for me to adequately explain what was motivating my change. Most of my friends were not in the health sciences profession and had not been trained in physiology or metabolism. Even though most people have a basic understanding that eating sugar is unhealthy, it's hard to conceive of the magnitude of cellular damage resulting from excess carbohydrates unless you've spent a good amount of time studying it (or suffering from it, which you may do if you're diabetic). Basic schooling fails to teach us how the body works, what our organs do, or how food is metabolized. If you got a superficial semester on the subject in high school, then you're one of the lucky ones. If you want to learn how your body does the very important work of turning your food into energy to fuel your cells and literally keep you running, you'll have to study the subject in college, or at least do some extracurricular reading.

Back in grad school, when I was quickly shrinking from lack of carbs, I faced one of the biggest challenges a low-carb dieter will ever face: pressure from my primary care physician to eat just like everyone else. (Never mind that such a diet could lead to weight gain and diabetes!) My doctor did a quick physical exam and declared me too thin. She asked about my diet, and I told her I'd chosen to eat only whole foods and mostly stay away from starch and sugar. She barely listened to me and didn't inquire as to why I'd made this shift. She just told me to gain weight. I was embarrassed and intimidated, and a week later, I quit my "diet." I was surprised at how quickly I caved under social pressure, and how easily I was convinced that something that felt right for me was actually doing me harm. But maybe it's because I *wanted* to believe that it was okay to eat lots of sugary foods that I let myself be persuaded to give up my abstinence. And, just like that, I went right back to eating all the sugar and starch I wanted—which was a lot. My appetite for sweets, like that of a lot of people I know, is insatiable. I'd gladly eat dessert every day if I had the opportunity. My taste buds want to, but my education in nutrition and my experience working with people who are overweight and struggling with poor health pleads with me not to. When sweets are in the picture, it's a constant battle.

My Ketogenic Diet Experiment

When the offer came to write this book I was already back to eating a much lower-carb diet than the average person. It had been almost a decade since my doctor's warning had pushed me off the low-carb wagon, and I'd regained some control over my sweet tooth. I'd completely eliminated gluten and most sources of sugar, and I was contemplating my next step. I'm not sure I would have delved fully into the ketogenic diet if not for the motivation of this book. I didn't have weight to lose, so I might have stopped just short of ketogenic, having carb-heavy foods maybe 20 percent of the time and never knowing how freeing a ketogenic diet could be. But since I like to experiment, I took the project and set myself up for four months of ketogenic life.

For the first two months I kept my carbs at or below 20 g per day and lost 9 lbs. After two months I started to add carbs back in until I was at about 50 g per day, which seemed like a huge amount! In contrast to the lower level, this new, bigger allotment of carbs made me feel like I could pretty much eat anything I wanted to. And I didn't really want much. I was really no longer interested in bread or anything made with flour, and very sweet foods like cookies and chocolate seemed intolerable to me. My taste buds had changed what they craved. I'd never been a big fan of potatoes, but meals based on rice and beans are a part of my cultural heritage, and I find it unnatural to dismiss my roots. I can imagine having some of these foods again when nostalgia hits (though to be honest, right now just the thought of eating a plateful of grains and legumes makes my belly feel uncomfortably full). Aside from the foods that link me emotionally to family and culture, I am surprised to discover that I don't miss many of the less meaningful (but quite tasty) foods I was initially afraid to give up.

After two months on my ketosis-sustaining allotment of carbs I just didn't really care about indulging in ice cream or having a bowl of pasta. I wasn't craving much of anything, actually. I was completely satisfied with my meals and rarely ever felt hungry. It was a welcome freedom I don't recall having often in my adult life.

Now that I've experienced life on the ketogenic diet I realize that the thing I like most about having carbohydrates in my diet is having some sweet elements to use in my cooking. Sweet is one of the four basic flavors (the others are sour, salty, and bitter, and the "meaty" flavor of umami is sometimes considered a fifth), so eliminating it completely lessens the spectrum of flavor in my cooking. I like adding a touch of sugar to my tomato sauce, or honey to a lemon vinaigrette to balance some of the acidity. The good news is that although I did forego these ingredients during the first months when I kept my carbs below 20 g, I was able to put them back in as soon as I bumped up to 50 g because they are used in small amounts and didn't put my meals over the edge.

Are You a Cheater?

Some people ask me if I really stuck to the diet the whole time. The answer is yes, I did. I only once considered cheating outright. I was scheming to have a chef friend create an elaborate, multi-course birthday dinner for a dear friend who was not on the ketogenic diet. I planned to eat all the courses along with him, including whatever rice, potatoes, breading, or sugar the dishes contained. I didn't go through with it, though. I just wanted to stick to my commitment, so I took my friend to eat somewhere else. And to be honest, at the time I couldn't even imagine eating what I knew would be a seven- or eight-course meal. Most of the time on the ketogenic diet I felt comfortably sated with small portions of food and didn't think much about my next meal until it arrived.

Although I never cheated consciously, it did take me a while to figure out that kale had seven times as many net carbs as any other green leafy thing I might use as the base of a salad. When I figured that out I made the switch to arugula and spinach, which didn't eat up my carb allotment so quickly! Perhaps I should mention here that, contrary to popular belief, nutritionists do not have memorized the exact nutrient amounts of every edible item on the planet! We know roughly how many calories are in many, many foods, and we know the proportion of macronutrients and key vitamins and minerals in commonly eaten foods. But just like physicians may use a desk reference to check the exact dose of a prescription, dietitians refer to a nutrient database when we need to know the exact nutrient content of a given food

So you can imagine my excitement when, in week four of my diet, I looked up the carb content of red wine and discovered that five ounces has only 5 g of net carbs. Although I rarely drink alcohol, this was cause for celebration! I had a nice glass of vino that very night. Diet or not, sometimes you've got to treat yourself!

Counting on Keto

During the first phase of the diet I was preoccupied with counting carbs. I was just worried all the time about the little bit of carbs in all of the keto-friendly foods I was eating. For example, I worried that the two or three grams each from my walnuts or celery or avocado would bring me out of ketosis. And then I took myself out of the seat of dieter and into that of scientist and realized: you don't have to be constantly worried about ruining your ketogenic state. Metabolism is a dynamic process. If you eat too many carbs one day you will slow ketone production for a little while, and then when you get back below your carb threshold ketone production will resume. It's not the sort of thing that requires absolute precision. You can't control what's in everything you eat, and if you try, it can make you crazy. For me, the key was eliminating foods that are mainly starch or sugar (e.g., apples and sweet potatoes) and getting a handle on the carb content of the few dozen foods I ate most often. Data on food consumption show that people eat about thirty different foods on a regular basis, cycling through them all in about four days. I'd say that's about right for me. So I learned to eyeball carb counts in those foods, and after a few weeks I was able to relax and stop obsessing about counting every bite.

Gratitude for Food

People often asked me if I felt deprived on the diet. Honestly, it was hard for me to feel sorry for myself when I considered that so many others face real hunger every single day. According to the United Nations World Food Programme (WFP), 842 million people in the world do not have enough to eat. I have been really fortunate that, for all of my life, I have never *truly* experienced hunger. I've always been able to get the food I need and want. Even though I'm normal weight, I'm one of the "overfed" when it comes to global comparisons. So while I sometimes missed the taste of certain things on the ketogenic diet, I wasn't exactly left *wanting*. Here I was, eating a variety of rich, healthful foods, and doing it so that I could publish a useful book and look better in my skinny jeans. What did I have to complain about?

I think one of the reasons dieting is a challenge is that we often take food for granted. It is all around us—with the least healthful types being the cheapest and most accessible— and so we indulge. A few years ago, I lived and worked on a coffee farm in Hawaii. Although we didn't grow food on a large scale, there was food on the farm. The chickens laid eggs, and an avocado tree outside my window provided more avocados than we could ever eat. A macadamia tree grove and dozens of mango trees gave me plentiful access to foods that had always been a rare and exotic treat before. The grocery store was far away, so we planned food needs in advance and made do with whatever else fell from the sky (or the chicken's bottom). One night we killed a wild pig.

He had fattened himself on avocados and macadamia nuts, and when we ate him we participated mindfully in the cycle of life that feeds us all. I held a deep respect that evening for the animal whose life had been sacrificed so that I could be nourished. It felt much different to eat that way, and I felt a deep gratitude for the food before me—much more so than I usually feel for the foods I grab thoughtlessly off the grocery store shelf in my typical urban surroundings. It's easier there to forget how valuable the food really is—how it represents years of soil and sunlight that nourish a tree that grows heavy with avocados which fall to feed a pig that ultimately may nourish you.

Eating on a ketogenic diet helped me slow down and be more thoughtful with my meals. Perhaps I was able to do so because when I removed sugar and starch I also got rid of the intense feeling of needing to eat the very moment I felt a twinge of hunger. I didn't have the drive toward food that used to come when my blood sugar would cycle up and down on a carb-heavy diet. When I would get hungry on that type of diet, nothing would get between me and my meal! But the ketogenic diet made me a bit more civilized with my eating tendencies and helped me remember that I am fortunate for having all the food I need every day of my life.

CHAPTER 1

Overview of the Ketogenic Diet

What is it? Where does it come from?
Is it safe? Who's using it today?

What Is the Ketogenic Diet?

The ketogenic diet has gotten a lot of criticism over the years for being a diet where you basically eat bacon and butter all day long. "Even if you do lose weight," people say, "that just seems unhealthy!" It *is* unhealthy! And it's not a smart way to go about a ketogenic diet.

The ketogenic diet consists of a mix of high-quality fats and protein foods, like avocado, chicken, salmon, almonds, and olive oil, as well as non-starchy, vitamin-rich vegetables like broccoli, cauliflower, asparagus, spinach, lettuce, tomatoes, and mushrooms. So-called indulgences, like red meat, full-fat cheese, and egg yolks, are also allowed. The diet eliminates sugar, flour, starch, fried foods, sweetened beverages, and low-quality processed foods. This last part shouldn't come as a surprise to anyone familiar with nutrition: try losing weight while eating sugary, floury, fried foods! It's *not* a winning strategy.

The ketogenic diet is a clear-cut path to the healthful, whole foods diet that most diet books, nutritionists, and concerned physicians recommend. It is *not* an animal-based diet, nor is it a high-protein diet. It is a *fat-based diet*. Followers of the ketogenic diet must eat *a mix of fats from animal and plant sources*, as well as non-starchy vegetables and a moderate amount of protein, while avoiding nutrient-poor carbohydrates in the form of starches and sugars. This eating pattern sends a message to your cells that says, "Please use fat instead of carbs." Once this message is received, after a few days of keeping your carb intake below 25–50 g (100–200 calories) *at most*, you enter a new metabolic state called *ketosis*, which confirms that your body is fueling the majority of its energy needs with fat. Ketosis is the gateway to rapid fat loss, and carb control is the key to that gate. You keep the fat-burning metabolism turned on by keeping your carb intake low.

In addition to using more fat for energy on the ketogenic diet relative to other diets, ketosis is proposed to work in various other ways to speed up and increase weight loss, including:

- Suppressing appetite, so people automatically eat less;
- Requiring more energy for metabolic processes, so that resting energy expenditure is increased;
- Stabilizing blood sugar and lowering insulin levels, which reduces fat storage and diminishes hunger;
- Enhancing mood, which helps some people avoid emotional eating;

- Reducing food choice, so that there are fewer opportunities for eating; and

- Eliminating "trigger foods," so people have more control over their eating habits.

Ketogenic Weight Loss

Research attributes the consistent weight loss effects of the ketogenic diet to these and many other mechanisms. For now, it's important to understand that:

- The objective of the ketogenic diet is to achieve and maintain ketosis, the state in which you use mostly fat for energy;

- You do this by eating no more than 25–50 g of net carbs per day (some people can eat more and others need less); and

- You do not have to count calories or otherwise restrict your meals.

Despite the effectiveness of the ketogenic diet, many practitioners in the field are reluctant to use the term "ketogenic," or even suggest that their patients dramatically cut down on carbs. Perhaps they shy away from this approach because it goes against social norms. After all, most people eat a lot of carbs, don't they? It's expected of us. We live in a world full of sugar-laden, starch-filled goodies—muffins or cereal for breakfast, high-fructose corn syrup in salad dressings at lunch, sugary "energy bars" to snack on during the day, and dinner plates loaded with rice or potatoes. These foods are everywhere, and it's easy to munch on them mindlessly as we go about our business. We might even say they're a great convenience, because they provide a constant source of energy for very little effort on our part.

But these foods are not helping us. Instead, they're driving so much fat onto our bodies that we're riddled with diseases of metabolic dysfunction, such as diabetes, cardiovascular disease, and cancer. According to the Centers for Disease Control and Prevention (CDC), over one-third of US adults (78 million people) are obese. We are considered the second fattest nation in the world (Mexico recently knocked us out of first place)—and it's looking more and more likely that our obsession with carbohydrates is to blame. You don't have to follow the (overweight) crowd on this one. If you're serious about improving your health and living life at a comfortable weight, then you may want to carefully reconsider the role of sugar and starch in your diet. If you're ready to do that, the ketogenic diet may be just right for you.

The ketogenic diet is high in fat, moderate in protein, and very low in digestible carbohydrate (fiber is not restricted). You *don't* eat starchy foods like bread, rice, flour, oats, potatoes, or corn, or sweet foods like cakes, cookies, candy, most fruits, or desserts. You *do* eat nutritious, non-starchy vegetables, meats, poultry, fish, eggs, dairy, nuts, seeds, and oils. Very few of your calories come from carbohydrates, a small portion come from protein, and the majority come from fat.

Fat! You may be thinking: *But everyone knows that you have to cut down on fat if you want to lose weight! Every diet I've ever done has advised steering clear of fat.* Ah, is that so? Well if that strategy worked so well, *then why are you still dieting?*

It turns out that eating fat doesn't make you fat, exactly. It's closer to the truth to say that *eating sugar* makes you fat.

Or, that eating sugar leads to *overeating* sugar (because sugar is so yummy and also because it's in everything, everywhere), which leads to chronically high blood sugar and insulin levels, which make you fat. And since all carbohydrates turn into sugar by the time they reach your bloodstream, well...you get the picture.

It's not clear that cutting down on fat will slim you. But *cutting down on carbohydrates*—way down—will almost certainly do the trick.

This is not a new idea. The role of carbohydrates in weight gain and loss has been well understood for centuries. The French gastronome Jean Brillat-Savarin wrote in 1825, in his famous book *The Physiology of Taste*, that one of the causes of obesity "is the fact that [starch] matter is the basis of our daily food."[1] This starchy matter is "more prompt in its action," he says, "when it is mingled with sugar." This should come as no surprise, the Frenchman said, since the standard practice for fattening farm animals is to feed them starch, and, surely, humans eating such a diet will quickly become fat as well. His proposed cure for obesity was to avoid "white rolls...biscuits...cakes...all the good things made with sugar...and farina.... [To eat] neither potatoes nor macaroni...," and so on.

In 1864, a wealthy and obese British man named William Banting wrote *Letter on Corpulence, Addressed to the Public*. In it, he described the starch-and-sugar-restricted diet that helped him lose 46 lbs in one year. Banting published and distributed the pamphlet for free, "desirous of circulating [his] humble knowledge and experience for the

---

1   Brillat-Savarin used "farinaceous" and "feculaferous" to mean "starch," but those terms are not well understood today.

benefit of [his] fellow man." Obesity, he said, was poorly understood, and he thought the cures recommended by physicians at the time were useless, as they had not helped him shed any pounds. Banting had been saved from a lifetime of obesity by the simple act of cutting out bread, sugar, beer, and potatoes, and he wanted to do the good deed of sharing this highly effective, yet seemingly unknown, weight-loss solution widely.

More recently, in 1972, Dr. Robert C. Atkins, a physician who had also had personal weight loss success with carbohydrate restriction, published *Dr. Atkins' Diet Revolution*. The book was the first to explain ketogenic metabolism (and the superior weight loss effects of ketosis) to a broad audience; it instantly sold millions, and, together with the later edition (*Dr. Atkins' New Diet Revolution*, in 1992), made the notion of carbohydrate restriction for weight loss familiar to the late-twentieth-century public. Through the '80s and '90s the diet was wildly popular, and very-low-carb eating became synonymous with "Atkins." Followers reported great success (who among us hasn't heard of someone who lost weight on the Atkins diet?) Again, as in centuries before, we saw that the sugar-and-starch-restricted diet worked. (See page 249 for a more detailed discussion of the Atkins diet.)

Why does this diet work so well? When you eat very few carbohydrates, your body changes the way it metabolizes nutrients. You begin using the fat stored in your cells for energy instead of using that blueberry muffin you ate for breakfast. Of course your body uses *some* fat for energy anytime you haven't eaten for a while, but in that situation you're likely *hungry*, which prompts you to eat, which shuts down the fat-burning machinery. You toggle back and forth between the fat-burning state and the carbohydrate-burning state, and, just when you're deep into the fat burning groove, you eat some carbs, which locks those fats right back up in your fat cells. It's a one step forward, two steps back sort of process—one in which you may lose weight, or you may *gain* it, depending on how good your body is at burning or storing energy. Or, you may just become frustrated with the whole business (rightly so) and decide to eat a candy bar.

The experience of being on the ketogenic diet is a very different one. The ketogenic diet *shifts the body entirely to an alternate state of metabolism*, so that you never swing back to using carbs for energy. Your body burns fat and... more fat. It burns fat when you're eating and not eating; it burns fat when you're sleeping, sitting, standing, reading, and exercising. As long as you avoid carbohydrates, your body continuously burns fat. (Oh, and you're rarely hungry on the ketogenic diet, so you will probably eat less as a side effect—which is a nice bonus for anyone with a busy life who'd rather not waste time looking for meals morning, noon, and night.) The are a number of other benefits to the ketogenic diet in addition to relatively rapid fat loss, including improved mood, increased energy level, and greater mental clarity. The rest of this book will explain why the ketogenic diet suppresses hunger and dissolves fat cells, tell you how to follow the diet for successful weight loss, and, ultimately, achieve better living and good health through carbohydrate restriction.

But wait, you're thinking. *Do I have to get rid of all high-carbohydrate foods? Can't I just have my sandwich on one slice of bread and eat muffins only on the weekends?* Well, you could do that, and if you're currently eating muffins every day for breakfast and sandwiches for lunch, that approach will probably knock off a few pounds. Assuming you're overweight, that's a good thing. If you cut down on starch and sugar you'll be moving in the right direction. You'll slowly begin to lose weight, and the quality of your diet will greatly improve. You won't get the benefits of ketosis, which means that you will probably be stuck with hunger and cravings a lot of the time. But if all you're ready to do is cut out a slice of daily bread and quit eating morning pastries, then go for it! After a month or two you'll become aware of which foods are high in carbohydrates, so you can eat less of them—and, if you stay away from sugar, your sugar cravings will diminish or disappear altogether. You may decide at that time that you're ready to go full-on with the ketogenic diet and quickly lose the extra weight. Whether or not you commit now to the ketogenic diet or just decide to cut down on desserts as a start is up to you. It depends on how much weight you have to lose and how fast you want to lose it. If you want to lose weight quickly without hunger, the ketogenic diet offers you that option.

Despite this, the ketogenic diet has not been promoted as an effective weight-loss tool by health or nutrition experts. For the most part, in fact, it's been discouraged. Nutritional guidance over the last few decades strongly advised Americans to avoid eating fat or—despite a lack of evidence to support the claim—risk gaining weight and developing heart disease. So we avoided buttering our bread and ate a lot of low-fat cookies and cakes in which the fat was replaced with added sugar. But we didn't lose weight (actually, we got fatter), nor did we collectively prevent heart disease (it's still the leading cause of death in the United States today). This particular story is more about politics than it is about nutrition and health, and it has been written about in great detail elsewhere. The book *Good Calories, Bad Calories*, by the well-known science journalist Gary Taubes, covers the history in detail, as do a number of other books and news articles published in the last decade. If you've any interest in the bigger story you have only to do a quick news search to find headlines like the following:

- A Call for a Low-Carb Diet That Embraces Fat. *New York Times*, September 1, 2014
- Ending the War on Fat. *Time Magazine*, June 23, 2014
- Study Questions Fat and Heart Disease Link. *New York Times*, March 17, 2014
- What Really Makes Us Fat? *New York Times*, June 30, 2012
- Diet and Fat: A Severe Case of Mistaken Consensus. *New York Times*, October 9, 2007
- What If It's All Been a Big Fat Lie? *New York Times*, July 7, 2002

The most recent of these appeared in 2014, just as I was writing this book, and nearly every day now there seems to be another story suggesting that our outlook on fat is changing. Allow the nation's top nutrition experts at Harvard's School of Public Health to sum it up for you:

> It's time to end the low-fat myth. For decades, a low-fat diet was touted as a way to lose weight and prevent or control heart disease and other chronic conditions, and food companies re-engineered products to be reduced-fat or fat-free, often compensating for differences in flavor and texture by increasing amounts of salt, sugar, or refined grains. However, as a

*nation, following a low-fat diet hasn't helped
us control weight or become healthier.*[2]

In other words, following the advice they were given, Americans cut down significantly on fat intake—from 45 percent of calories in the 1960s, to 33 percent of calories today—effectively removing *one-quarter* of the fat from their diets; and yet, over the same time period, almost *three times* as many people became obese, and more than *ten times* as many people developed diabetes.

Yikes! The statistics can really make you wonder: If people aren't eating a lot of fat, what on earth are they eating? Carbohydrates, by the truckload. According to national diet survey data, men consume about 1,300 calories from carbohydrates per day (out of a daily total of 2,700), and women average about 950 calories from carbohydrates per day (out of a daily total of 1,850).[3] That's *half* of daily calories from carbs! Think about the foods you eat on a regular basis. If you're eating like the average person, these foods are mostly made of flour, sugar, and starch. When I ask my clients for diet records I see this trend: egg whites, dry toast, coffee with many sugars, low-fat flavored yogurt, reliance on pasta and sandwiches for lunch, a lot of energy bars, and avoidance of steak and avocado. Every one of them is overweight.

The Harvard researchers go on to remind us that fat is an essential nutrient, which is why it appears in small amounts

---

2   The Nutrition Source, "Fats and Cholesterol: Out with the Bad, In with the Good," Harvard School of Public Health. Last accessed on September 2, 2014. http://www.hsph.harvard.edu/nutritionsource/fats-full-story.

3   According to data from the national survey, "What We Eat in America," men eat an average of 322 g (1288 kcal) of carbohydrates per day, and women average 237 g (948 kcal) per day.

in almost all foods. "Even quintessential fat-free foods like carrots and lettuce," they say, contain fat. "That's a testament to how important fats are for life." They wrap up by saying:

> It is a common belief that the more fat you eat, the more weight and body fat you gain. This belief has been bolstered by much of the nutritional advice given to people over the past few decades, which has focused on lowering total fat intake while increasing carbohydrate intake. But the notion that food fat equals body fat isn't completely true, and the advice has been misguided.

Wow. That's big news! So if not eating fat makes you fat, does eating fat make you thin?

First, it's important to understand that a high-fat diet is by definition a low-carb diet,[4] *but not all low-carb diets are ketogenic.* A diet must be very low in carbohydrates to be ketogenic (also called very-low-carbohydrate ketogenic diet, or VLCKD).

Second, it's important to understand how different groups seek to answer this question.

Scientific researchers often do controlled experiments. They take groups of volunteers, put them on different types of diets (a high-fat, low-carb diet; or a low-fat, high-carb diet; or something else), and compare how much weight each group loses. When those in the low-carb group lose more, as they almost always do, researchers conclude that eating a high-fat, low-carb diet causes people to lose weight. Pub-

---

4   Conversely, a low-fat diet is necessarily high in carbs. Calories must come from somewhere, and I struggle to think of any healthful diet schemes that recommend eating a majority of calories from protein.

lic health researchers may review historical and population data (i.e., look at the trends in diet habits over time and compare them to weight changes over time), and draw conclusions about the effectiveness of low-fat or low-carb diets. Clinicians, such as doctors, dietitians, and other healthcare professionals who provide care directly to individuals, tend to observe what happens to their patients who use different strategies for weight loss. Inevitably, regardless of advice given, some people will try low-carb diets on their own (and others will try low-fat, and other types). When patients following a low-fat diet fail to lose weight and/or continue to gain it, as they often do, and those on a low-carb diet lose weight, as they almost always do, the healthcare provider concludes that eating a high-fat, low-carb diet is effective for weight loss.

Anyone who isn't professionally engaged in helping people lose weight can use their intuition and observations of real life to answer the question of whether high-fat, low-carb diets make you thin. A fantastic line written in the 1960s in the *British Journal of Nutrition* is commonly quoted in the low-carb community. It says simply, "Every woman knows that carbohydrate is fattening."

Have *you* personally ever tried a low-carb diet? I'll bet you lost weight. Have you ever noticed a friend who starts to leave the rice on her dinner plate, avoids the bread basket, and orders eggs instead of pancakes for breakfast? She loses weight, right? I am hard-pressed to think of an example of someone who followed a low-carb diet and *didn't* lose weight.

If you want to lose weight you have to meet two targets: a metabolic target and a behavioral target. Success will come when you make a meaningful change in a common behavior, something you do *all the time*, that's causing you to hold onto weight. Even in the world of low-fat dieting, doctors who tell overweight patients to stay away from bacon are really missing the point. *People don't eat bacon every day*! It takes too long to cook and clean up. People eat bacon once in a while, on a weekend. But you know what they eat every single day? Bread. And cereal, and potatoes, and sugar, and rice, and more bread. More importantly, bacon, made mostly of fat, doesn't cause a spike in blood sugar and insulin that demands that the body store more fat in fat cells. You know what does that? Bread, and its fat-free, carb-rich friends mentioned above. Nudging these foods out of your diet communicates to your body that you prefer to metabolize fat for fuel. You'll begin losing weight quickly (achieving your metabolic target), and you'll be astonished to see how a carb-heavy diet—despite what nutritional guidelines have led you to believe—has been strongly influencing your body to hold onto weight.

Times Are Changing

Thanks in part to good research, thoughtful communications, articles, books, and interviews from scientists, health-care professionals, and interested individuals who have made these observations themselves, there is something of a revolution underway in the world of nutrition. Carbohydrates are finally being properly blamed for their role in weight gain and disease, and fats are being exonerated. Progressive and outspoken physicians like Dr. Mark Hyman, author of *The Blood Sugar Solution*, Dr. David Perlmutter, author of *Grain Brain*, and Dr. William Davis, author of

Wheat Belly, are leading the change in the medical community. You'll notice that these and other health professionals who recommend carbohydrate-restricted diets in their work also tend to follow them in their personal lives. If you do an image search for any of the names listed above you'll notice they appear slim and in good health. It's hard not to believe that they're doing something right.

It's also helpful that the paleo diet, which promotes whole foods, embraces dietary fat, and denounces flour and sugar, is gaining in strength and numbers every day. Paleo is so popular that, whether intentional or not, it's driving a shift in societal thinking about the healthfulness of carbs and fats. In fact, a convenient way to explain your ketogenic diet to the uninitiated is to say, "You know the paleo diet? Well it's like the paleo diet on a diet. It's basically the same thing minus the desserts and sweet potatoes." What's more, while there are maybe only a dozen blogs or cookbooks devoted to the ketogenic diet, there are hundreds promoting the paleo diet—many sharing high-fat, low-carb recipes, and recommendations for food products suitable for the ketogenic dieter. The role of the paleo movement must be acknowledged, for without a change in social norms away from carbs and toward fats (as paleo is nudging things along) it would be much harder for an individual to stick to a high-fat diet plan.

The current groundswell of interest in and embrace of food fats will undoubtedly help you in your journey on the ketogenic diet. And while this is surely not the only path to weight loss, it is a highly effective one that's worth giving a try if you haven't managed to lose weight with low-fat diets. The ketogenic diet will prompt your body to burn fat for fuel. That's not a magic trick. It's your biology.

CHAPTER 2

The Ketogenic Diet Quick-Start Guide

If you're ready to dive into the ketogenic diet while still reading the book, this chapter is your guide. It covers what to eat, what not to eat, and what else to do to make your diet a success!

Unlocking a Treasure Trove of Energy

Have you ever had a well-meaning aunt or grandma give you a nice, crisp $100 bill? It's an exciting moment! That bill represents a lot of money. You start dreaming of the things you'll buy with it—then you carry the bill around in your wallet for weeks trying to use it, failing every time. You're late for work one morning and desperate for a cup of coffee, but the coffee shop won't accept such a large bill. You move on, grumpy and un-caffeinated, yet still over-rich. That night you go out to dinner with a friend. The meal costs $50 but the waitress can't break your hundred. You leave well-fed and still flush with cash—except that now you owe $25 to your friend. You're constantly aware that you have on you more money than you really need; but for various reasons, you can't seem to use it!

Like the holder of that $100 bill, you carry around with you much more energy than you need to fuel your daily activities. The body's fat cells store over 130,000 calories![5] Wouldn't it be great if you had easy access to that energy whenever you felt hungry? Imagine even a week of such freedom—not having to eat every few hours to drive away that gnawing sensation in your belly. It would be like your personal metabolic vending machine delivering candy bars (er, broccoli) to your cells to keep you nourished all day without your having to exert any effort to find food.

Your fat stores are like that $100 bill: They represent a whole lot of currency—if only you could use it.

What Can I Eat?

The ketogenic diet gives you ready access to that big pool of energy buried in your fat cells. Achieving ketosis is like finding a friendly cashier to break your hundred dollar bill: finally, the money flows easily! Once your metabolism adapts to ketosis you'll be drawing constantly on your fat stores, rather than switching back and forth between using fat and glucose (sugar) for energy. (On a non-ketogenic diet your body uses mainly glucose after a meal and mainly fat in the space between meals.)

Now that you know how the ketogenic diet causes fat loss—and you're sure you want to lose fat—let's get down to the nitty-gritty of what you can eat.

---

5   The average 145-pound man stores 15 g of triglycerides, or 135,000 calories.

Fats Are Encouraged

Most foods contain a mix of macronutrients (the food components that provide energy to the human body), but the majority of calories in a particular food tend to come from one of three. Accordingly, foods can be classified roughly as either fats, proteins, or carbs. The following foods are made up mostly of fat, and they will be your main source of calories on the ketogenic diet:

- Oils (e.g., olive oil, coconut oil, sesame oil)
- Fats in the flesh of fish and meat
- Avocado
- Nuts (e.g., walnuts, almonds, pecans)
- Seeds (e.g., pumpkin, flax, chia)
- Coconut meat (only unsweetened)
- Butter, cream, and cheese

In general, you may eat "as much as you want" of these foods. However, keep in mind that the more calories you take in from food, the less your body will need to take out of fat stores. So while there is no restriction on how much fat you can have, it is a good idea to eat until you are 80 percent full. Fat takes a few hours to fully digest, and you will not feel hungry for a long while after a keto meal.

Metabolically speaking, you will not stop ketosis by eating too much fat. However, you may slow your weight loss if you overindulge.

The body uses different types of fats for different purposes, and it's important to eat a mix of fats from a variety of sources. The categorization of fats into "good fats" (the unsaturated types founds largely in plants) and "bad fats" (the saturated type found in larger concentration in animal foods) is based on the notion that saturated fat causes heart disease. This theory is now believed to be flawed. Instead, excess carbohydrate consumption is emerging as a major culprit in elevating heart disease risk. This subject is discussed in greater detail in Chapter 3.

Proteins Are Important

Protein is used in the body for building and repair of muscle tissue, and for various enzymatic functions. Normally, your body spares protein for these purposes and does not use much for energy. It is important to eat enough protein to maintain lean body (muscle) tissue and healthy functioning of body systems. Weight loss on any type of diet may cause loss of some lean tissue, so it is especially important to eat sufficient, high-quality protein while losing weight. Protein sources on the ketogenic diet include the following:

- Meats (e.g., beef, pork, lamb, buffalo, venison)
- Poultry (e.g., chicken, turkey, duck, goose, quail)
- Fish (e.g., mackerel, salmon, trout) and shellfish[6] (e.g., shrimp, lobster, calamari)
- Eggs
- Tofu and tempeh
- Cheese, yogurt, nuts, and seeds contain smaller amounts of protein.

Remember, the ketogenic diet is *not* a high-protein diet; it is a high-fat, moderate-protein diet. High-protein diets are generally not recommended for people in good health, and too much protein can be problematic for the ketogenic dieter for the following reasons: protein causes a rise in

---

6   Unlike fish, shellfish contain a small amount of carbs. Count your carb intake from these foods.

insulin, which inhibits fat breakdown; protein (in the form of amino acids) is used in the body to make glucose, and too much of it can diminish or suspend ketosis; and, eating too many calories of any sort will slow or inhibit weight loss. That said, unless you insist on believing (falsely) that the ketogenic diet is a meat-based diet, you will likely not be in danger of overloading on protein. Furthermore, proteins are highly satiating, and it can be unpleasant, if not downright difficult, to overeat protein foods if you practice to stop eating when you are full. A moderately high amount of protein in the range of 1.2–1.7 g/kg[7] of body weight (81–115 g for someone weighing 150 lbs) is commonly used in studies of ketogenic diets with no ill effects and is a good range to aim for in your diet. You may use 2 g/kg (136 g for a 150-pound person) if you exercise frequently.

The protein content of foods varies somewhat with the type. For example, different cuts of meat have different amounts of protein, as do different types of fish. When possible, check the label of the specific food you're eating. Use these amounts as a general rule:

- Meat, poultry, and fish (including steak, chicken, salmon, sardines, lamb, veal, and ground beef) have about 24 g of protein per 3 oz.
  3 oz of meat is about the size of a deck of cards. 3 oz of fish is about the size of a checkbook.

- Hard cheeses have about 7 g per ounce (about the size of two dice).

- Eggs have about 7 g each.

---

7   The standard form of equations for protein and energy needs uses kilograms rather than pounds of body weight. One (1) kilogram (kg) = 2.2 pounds (lbs).

- Tofu has about 7 g and tempeh has about 15 g per 3 oz (the size of a deck of cards).
- Nuts have about 7 g per ounce (varies).

Net Carbohydrates

Throughout this book, the terms "carbohydrates" or "carbs" should be taken to mean net (or digestible) carbohydrates. The digestible forms of carbohydrate are starch and sugar. A third form of carbohydrate, fiber, is indigestible, and need not be restricted. This subject is addressed in further detail in Chapter 4.

Most Carbs Are Forbidden

This is the crux of the ketogenic diet! Do not under any circumstances eat any of the following foods:

- Things made with sugar or caloric sweeteners (e.g., honey, agave, maple syrup)
- Things made with flour (e.g., bread, pastries, pasta)
- Grains (e.g., rice, oats, quinoa, couscous)
- Fruit, except small amounts of very-low-sugar fruits (e.g., strawberries)
- Starchy vegetables (e.g., potatoes, sweet potatoes, corn, peas)
- Lactose-rich dairy products (e.g., milk, ice cream, most yogurts)

The list above isn't exhaustive. A more complete list of foods to avoid is given in Chapter 7. Be aware that many foods that seem low-carb or carb-free may contain "hidden" sugar. For example, tomato sauce and salad dressings often have sugar listed as an ingredient, and sweeteners are widely used in foods like beef jerky and deli meats. It is crucial to read food labels and count your net carbs. Keep carb intake to 25–50 g per day. If you eat too many carbs, you will stop ketosis and halt your diet.

Not All Carbs Are Created Equal

You *do* want to eat high-fiber, vitamin-and-mineral-rich, low-calorie carbohydrate foods. Most of these are non-starchy vegetables like spinach, kale, broccoli, cauliflower, cucumber, tomatoes, asparagus, peppers, onions, mushrooms, and the list goes on. These should make up the bulk of your carb intake. You may also eat a small amount of berries (e.g., strawberries, blueberries), but don't overdo it—since these foods have more carbs per serving than the others, you will use up your carb allotment more quickly on days that you eat them.

What Else Do I Need to Do?

You have the basics now. The following tips will help you keep on the straight and narrow. You must:

Understand that you don't need carbs. Since you've been eating carbohydrates your whole life, you might be wondering if it's okay to cut them out more or less completely. Surprising as it may be, we don't need to get carbohydrates from our diet! It turns out that our bodies can make all the carbohydrate we need. This is not true of fats, protein, many vitamins, minerals, water, or fiber. If we don't get these nutrients from our diet, we develop deficiency diseases and eventually die. If we don't get carbohydrates from our diet, after a while we just...stop getting fat.

Don't be afraid of fat. If you are scared to eat fat you will not succeed on the ketogenic diet. This may be a challenge for some people, because dietary advice has discouraged fat for some time. This is unfortunate. Eating fat will likely not give you heart disease or make you overweight (but eating carbohydrates very well might). Fat is the foundation of the ketogenic diet. If you need to do some self-directed mind changing to get yourself out of the "fat is bad" mode, do that before you start the diet. Read Chapter 3 "Fat in All Its Forms" to help you along.

Count your carbs. Do not assume that you know the carb content of any food. Use the lists in Chapter 7 "What Can I Eat?" to get a handle on fresh foods, and ALWAYS read the nutrition facts on packaged foods. The net carb content of a food is the amount of total carbohydrate minus the amount of fiber.

Drink plenty of water. Ketogenic diets promote water loss, and dehydration can cause fatigue and general malaise. Pay attention to your thirst cues and be diligent about drinking water. Drink more if you're also consuming caffeine, sweating, or living in a hot climate.

Supplement sodium and electrolytes. The kidneys excrete more sodium during ketosis, and an imbalance of electrolytes can make you feel ill. Make an effort to add salt to foods, and drink high-quality broth when available. Take a multivitamin that includes potassium and magnesium as well.

Eat when you're hungry and stop when you're full. The diet will get rid of your cravings and greatly diminish your hunger. Let it do its job! If you're a mindless eater who pays little attention to hunger cues and can eat huge amounts of food even when you're full, then it's probably a good idea to reshape that behavior sooner rather than later so you can reap the full benefits of the ketogenic diet. The exercises in Chapter 5 will help you in this regard.

Ask for the ingredients in everything. If you're neither a food professional nor a big fan of cooking, then you may not know the ingredients in a lot of the foods you eat that are prepared by others. Just ask. You'll be surprised at how many sauces include flour or sugar, how often fish is lightly floured before being baked, etc.

Make a commitment to yourself and your diet. Research on "behavior change" (in which eating habits are a popular category of inquiry) suggests that people who identify specific goals and commit to them explicitly are more likely to achieve them than those who have a vague notion of what they want to achieve. For example, "I commit to eating less than 50 g of carbs per day for at least 60 days, and if I have not reached my goal weight I will extend my commitment 30 days at a time until I have lost 25 lbs" is more effective than "I'm going to follow a ketogenic diet to lose weight." Describing a detailed behavior (eating less than 50 g of carbs per day), a time frame (at least 60 days), and a conditional next step (extending the commitment 30 days at a time until goal weight is reached) is essential. Putting your commitment in writing or stating it out loud to someone else will further increase chances of success.

Now that you've gotten the list of "musts," you would be foolish not to:

Keep some favorite keto foods around. Do some exploration at the grocery store and get a bunch of things that fit into the diet. Almond butter, flax crackers, full-fat cheese, seaweed snacks, and nuts are good options. As you progress on the ketogenic diet you won't feel much like snacking, but in the beginning, as you're changing your eating habits, you want to give yourself an array of options to assure you'll stick with it.

Get rid of the foods in your kitchen that are not allowed. I have a lot of clients who tell me they'll start their diet after they finish the _____ in their kitchen because, as they learned as a child at the dinner table, there are hungry people in the world, so they hate throwing food away. I can relate to that viewpoint. That's why, when I started the ketogenic diet, I gave all my rice, sugar, ice cream, maple syrup, and raisins to a friend. You can pack the stuff up and drop it off at a local food pantry if you prefer. Just don't use it as an excuse to ease slowly into the diet. Ketogenic is all in or all out. Getting rid of the stuff will make it a whole lot easier to jump onboard.

Pick four or five keto-friendly meals that you really like. And plan to make them weekly. This is a key element in any healthy eating plan. People tend to eat the same foods week after week, and having a handful of favorite dishes to choose from will help you avoid the otherwise inevitable weekday evening panic of "What's for dinner?" It's better not to get caught without a clue as to what to eat. Take some time to peruse the recipe section of this book (page 271), or even pick out some keto-friendly recipes from cookbooks or recipe sites you use now. This will give you a stable foundation on which to build your new eating habits.

Take a fiber supplement. Since you've read the food guidelines above I know you'll be eating a lot of fresh vegetables and drinking a lot of water on your diet, right? Vegetables (and to a lesser extent nuts and seeds) contain soluble and insoluble fiber, both of which are important to good health. Soluble fiber helps you feel full, reduces blood sugar levels and insulin response, and reduces low-density lipoprotein (LDL) (or what some call "bad") cholesterol (the relationship of cholesterol to health is discussed more fully on page 44). Insoluble fiber tends to speed up bowel movements and prevent constipation. Most people don't get enough dietary fiber (the recommendation is 25 g/day for women and 38 g/day for men), and constipation is a widespread problem. Low-carb diets can increase risk for constipation because some fiber-containing foods, like fruits and whole grains, are absent on the diet. If you already struggle with constipation or you begin to on the diet, take a fiber supplement. You can find these in any drugstore, grocery store, or supplement shop. And drink more water!

Exercise. It should go without saying that exercise is essential to good health and helpful, if not required, for weight loss. Regardless of your eating pattern, regular exercise should be a part of your life! Among other things, exercise helps prevent heart disease, cancer, and diabetes, improves lung capacity, keeps bones strong, increases muscle strength, reduces depression and anxiety, improves mood, enhances cognitive function, prevents weight gain, and extends lifespan. Unless you are physically unable to exercise, it is absolutely a healthy and worthwhile endeavor. Unfortunately, many of us don't get enough—or even a little—exercise. Even worse, *many people believe that it's not possible to exercise on a ketogenic diet.* This is entirely false! You can absolutely exercise on a ketogenic diet. Doing so will help you lose weight faster and maintain muscle mass. Two key points: 1) include strengthening/weight training activities (not just aerobics) in your exercise regimen, and 2) for the first week or maybe two of the diet you will be transitioning to a fat-based metabolism and you may be too fatigued to exercise; that's okay, just wait until it passes and pick up the activity!

Finally, you might consider:

Starting your diet with a fast. Fasting for two to three days (48–72 hours) will help use up the sugar stores in your body and move you more quickly into ketosis. If you choose to fast, eat no food, but be sure to drink water (8–10 cups per day).

Checking your urine for ketones. At least, in the beginning. Ketones are the breakdown product of fats that your brain uses (instead of sugar) for energy on the ketogenic diet. You can buy ketone urine strips (or "ketostix") at any drugstore. They're either behind the pharmacy counter or shelved near the products for diabetics, and they cost $5–$10 for fifty strips. These give a crude estimate of the ketones in your urine and are not an accurate measure of blood ketone levels, nor will they tell you how much fat you're "burning." Still, especially in the beginning, it can be motivating to know that you're in ketosis at all (before you start the diet you should have no measurable ketones in your urine). Also, as you're beginning to learn the carb contents of various foods you may accidentally eat something with sugar or starch. In that case, you can measure your urine ketones and make note of how you feel (hunger cues, level of fatigue, clarity of thinking, gastrointestinal, or "GI," symptoms) when you're not in ketosis versus when you are; this information will be helpful later on for you to determine the level of carbs to eat for long-term weight maintenance.

Developing an eating-out game plan. It's easy to fall off a new diet the moment you're in an unfamiliar eating situation and have no idea what to choose. Rather than risk this deer-in-headlights scenario, sit down and think about the various places in which you're likely to eat in the next few weeks. Picture the office cafeteria, the dinner party at a friend's house next week, or the restaurant where you'll dine with clients on Friday night. The likelihood is that *these places will have options that fit in your diet*, although you may have to make some modifications (like swapping oil and vinegar for a raspberry vinaigrette on your salad). Either way, you will feel much calmer and be better equipped for success if you take some time to check out the cafeteria serving line before the lunch rush, have a conversation with your friend about your food restrictions, and peruse the restaurant menu online before you arrive.

Tracking your food intake. This is exceedingly easy nowadays, as we have a world of online and mobile diet-tracking apps to choose from. These allow you to enter the foods you eat and keep track of calories and nutrient intake. This could be very helpful to you in determining how many carbs you've eaten for the day, and thus staying within your carb allotment.

Taking a basic cooking class. Cooks know how to make food taste good without relying on sugar, which is an art that's somewhat lost in our processed and packaged food society. If you can't cook more than a pot of boiling water, a basic cooking class will give you a foundation to cook more of your own (and thus healthier) meals. Also, learning how to make certain dishes will give you a better sense of what's in them when you're eating out, which will help you avoid hidden carbs. If you're someone who knows your way around a kitchen, then you're likely already skilled in making your own sauces and marinades rather than getting them out of a jar, or in whipping up something other than pasta or rice as the main portion of a meal. Still, a lot of traditional cooking techniques take advantage of the flavor-enhancing properties of fat and salt—two ingredients deemed unhealthy in nutritional recommendations of the recent past. Luckily, the ketogenic diet encourages fat, and the physiologic changes that occur in ketosis require you to add more salt to your diet. So either dig out those old French cookbooks with the "heavy" dishes you long ago gave up, or take a class in traditional techniques. It will be an investment that will help you for the rest of your (hopefully low-carb) life.

CHAPTER 3

Fat in All Its Forms

If You're Not Eating Fat, What Are You Eating?

Most of my clients who are carrying excess weight (especially around their midsection) and struggling with the beginnings of diabetes and cardiovascular disease tend to eat the following things for breakfast:

- Plain toast, no butter, with a bowl of fruit
- Cereal and low-fat milk
- Waffles with "lite" maple syrup
- Egg white and low-fat cheese on a croissant with orange juice from a fast food restaurant
- Oatmeal with brown sugar and raisins
- Muffin or Danish and coffee with cream and sugar
- Fruit-flavored low-fat yogurt and granola
- A bagel with cream cheese and a banana

Do you notice a theme? These breakfasts are almost exclusively carbohydrate, and they are not ideal—especially for the type of person described above. This person has what's called "metabolic syndrome" (also known as insulin resistance syndrome, or syndrome X), a cluster of symptoms that appear together when the body can no longer handle the strain of a poor diet, excess weight, and lack of exercise. A person with metabolic syndrome is twice as likely to develop heart disease, and five times as likely to develop diabetes, as someone who doesn't have metabolic syndrome.

Having three of the following signs indicate the presence of metabolic syndrome:

- A large waist circumference (35 inches or more for women and 40 inches or more for men)
- A high triglyceride level (150 mg/dL[8] or higher)
- A low HDL (good cholesterol) level (less than 50 mg/dL for women and less than 40 mg/dL for men)
- High blood pressure (130/85 mmHg[9] or higher)
- High fasting blood sugar (100 mg/dL or higher)

Weight loss is key to reducing (or eliminating) the signs of metabolic syndrome, and thus lowering the risk of disease. Unfortunately, it is especially difficult for someone with insulin resistance, a major component of metabolic syndrome, to lose weight. That's because this person's cells have nearly stopped responding to insulin's signal to "take up" glucose from the bloodstream. Glucose can't remain in the blood for too long; it *must* move into cells and be metabolized for energy, or severe illness, and ultimately death, will occur. The body knows this, so it produces more and more insulin in an attempt to force cells to take up glucose, all the while making them less and less responsive (i.e., more "resistant") to insulin in normal amounts. Insulin

---

8   Milligrams per deciliter (mg/dL) are the units used to measure triglycerides, cholesterol, and blood sugar (also called blood glucose).

9   Millimeters of mercury (mmHg) are the units used to measure blood pressure.

also prevents the body from using fat, and actually causes it to make more! When a person with insulin resistance eats carbohydrates, their cells becomes even less responsive to insulin, and their body stores even more fat. The cycle of fat gain and increasing insulin resistance is self-perpetuating. Needless to say, weight loss for this person is quite difficult. (The effect of insulin on fat metabolism is discussed in detail on page 82.)

Many of my clients have metabolic syndrome, and they often consume a lot of high-carbohydrate foods like those listed above. They stick to these low-fat foods because they have been following misguided dietary advice about how to avoid gaining weight and getting heart disease. Unfortunately, this tactic has led them to grow fat bellies and dampen their cells' response to insulin, moving them all the time closer to the chronic diseases they so fear.

I spend a good deal of time undoing my clients' fears of fat. One woman, we'll call her Gisele, told me guiltily one day that she had had toast with nothing on it for breakfast that morning. I asked her which macronutrient was in toast. She said "fat," and looked ashamedly down at her feet. I asked her to try again. She looked confused. "Carbs?" she answered. "Yes, carbs!" I said. Gisele asked: "No fat? Are you sure?" I was sure. Gisele looked very happy until she noticed the alarm on my face. "You have diabetes," I said. "Carbs are very dangerous for you, *especially* if you eat them alone, without protein or fat, so that your blood sugar and insulin spike." The frustrating part is that Gisele was depriving herself of foods she loved in an effort to eat what she thought was a healthy diet, and replacing them with foods that were making her disease worse.

Over time, Gisele began to understand that all the carbs she was eating were causing her harm, and she adjusted her diet. She was able to bring back in things that she liked, including meat dishes from her traditional Mexican cuisine, whole milk, and whole eggs. She kept tortillas to a minimum, and completely quit drinking soda and juice. Her weight dropped, and so did her Hemoglobin A1C, a marker for blood glucose levels. This meant that Gisele was no longer walking around with too much sugar in her blood, and that maybe she'd have a chance to make use of some of the fat stored in her body in between meals.

If your breakfasts resemble the list above, or if you're perfectly comfortable eating slice after slice of bread at the dinner table but wouldn't dare touch the butter, then you may have a fear of fat. If this is you, you're certainly not alone. Nutritional guidance has long cautioned us to stay away from fat or risk getting fat, not to mention ending up with some terrible diseases; and worse, diet advice has given carbs a free pass. Many have the idea embedded firmly in their heads that carbs are totally harmless, and they can be eaten as much as is desired with no ill effects—including weight gain. Unfortunately, this is entirely untrue!

The relentless diet advice to stay away from fat in recent decades has understandably scared a lot of people off of butter, eggs, and even olive oil. It's no easy thing to go against the grain, especially when you think you may be doing yourself harm. Even some well-known authors who've written about the "fat controversy" of our generation—the mistaken belief that fat causes weight gain and heart disease, and the subsequent advice to avoid it and fill your plate instead with carbs—have said that as they uncovered the research that cleared fat's good name, they would still sometimes look down at their plate of bacon and eggs and wonder if they were harming themselves. It can be somewhat intimidating to follow a high-fat, low-carb diet when nearly every physician and nutritionist in the country is telling you that you're destroying your heart with every bite.

If you take away only one thing from this book, take the new understanding that fat is not your mortal enemy. If you struggle to eat a high-fat meal without fear that you're doing your body harm, I urge you to take a proactive approach to getting over this fear. Staying away from fat and replacing it with foods high in sugar and starch does you much more harm than good.

From the Harvard School of Public Health Nutrition Source:

> When people cut back on fat, they often switch to foods full of easily digested carbohydrates—white bread, white rice, potatoes, sugary drinks, and the like—or to fat-free products that replace healthful fats with sugar and refined carbohydrates. The body digests these carbohydrates very quickly, causing blood sugar and insulin levels to spike. Over time, eating lots of "fast carbs" can raise the risk of heart disease and diabetes as much as—or more than—eating too much saturated fat.

There is great variation in the quality of carbohydrate foods and their impact on blood sugar, disease risk, and overall health. Carbohydrates that digest slowly and contain a good amount of fiber, vitamins, and other nutrients (such as broccoli, brown rice, chickpeas, and grapefruit) are preferred to those we call "refined" (such as white bread, pasta, crackers, and soda), which digest quickly and tend to lack fiber and other nutrients. The ketogenic diet is more concerned with the amount of carbohydrate than the type; however, it's easy to see how taking the type of food into account can give a clue as to the amount of carbs it contains. In general, the carbs promoted on the ketogenic diet (mainly non-starchy vegetables) are slower to digest and more nutrient-rich than those that are prohibited (such as pasta and bread).

Not All Fats Are Created Equal

Recall that there are different types of fats found in foods. There are also different types of fats found in the body. There is widespread confusion and tremendous controversy regarding the relationship between food fats and health. The remainder of this chapter will focus on key points of understanding around fats, nutrition, and health.

Fats in Food

Most foods that are considered "fats" have a mix of three types: saturated, monounsaturated, and polyunsaturated. (Animal foods also have cholesterol, a fourth type of fat.) We often refer to foods by the type of fat they contain in the highest proportion. Saturated fats (SFA) are found mostly in animal products like meat, milk, and cheese, as well as coconut and palm oils. Monounsaturated fats (MUFA) are found in avocado, and in some nuts and plant oils, especially olive oil. Polyunsaturated fats (PUFA) are found in plant oils and grains, and a subset called the "essential fatty acids" are primarily found in fatty fish, and some nuts and seeds.

As we have discussed, the advice to avoid fats in general has been unwarranted with regard to health benefits and is particularly unhelpful when it comes to weight loss. It's more relevant to discuss the *type* of fat when it comes to health. Unsaturated fats like those found in olive oil and salmon are generally encouraged for good health, while saturated fats like those found in beef and eggs are considered part of a healthful diet or are discouraged, depending on the school of thought.

Cholesterol

It's useful to talk about cholesterol first for an important reason: when we talk about the impact of dietary fats on health, we are usually concerned with how they will affect cholesterol levels in the blood.

We consume cholesterol directly from foods like egg yolks, cheese, and other animal products. But the cholesterol in blood is influenced more by the mix of fats in the diet than by consumption of actual cholesterol from foods. Although we tend to think of cholesterol as a bad thing, that is not at all the case! Cholesterol is *essential to the body*. It's an important component of cell membranes, makes up a good portion of brain tissue, and is a building block for many hormones. Although we need cholesterol to live, we don't need to get it from food. The body can make cholesterol on its own out of either glucose or saturated fat. Whether you eat cholesterol or not, your liver is producing billions of cholesterol molecules every second.

When we talk about the role of cholesterol in health we are referring not to cholesterol itself but to molecules called "lipoproteins" (lipo = fat) that carry cholesterol and other fats through the blood. There are low-density lipoproteins (LDL), also known as the "bad" type of cholesterol, and high-density lipoproteins (HDL), also known as the "good" type cholesterol. This designation of good and bad is not entirely accurate. Although it was believed for some time that having more LDL in the blood raised a person's risk of heart disease, it is now understood that the size of the LDL particles is more important than the amount. Small, dense LDL particles are considered dangerous because they easily lodge in artery walls and cause inflammation that leads to heart disease, whereas light, fluffy LDL particles do not. The amounts and types of these particles is greatly influenced by diet and other lifestyle factors, as well as genetics.

Ready for the good news? Eating a lot of carbohydrates gives you more small, dense LDL particles that damage arteries and can lead to heart attacks. It is now understood that reducing carbohydrate intake can thus lower the risk of heart disease brought on by "bad" cholesterol. Eating more fat, including saturated fat, produces more of the big, fluffy LDL particles—the kind we want.

So what about the "good" cholesterol? Eating a lot of carbohydrates *lowers* the level of HDL, or "good" cholesterol, in the blood. And what do you think raises it? Yup: eating more fats, particularly MUFAs and PUFAs.

The bottom line is that cholesterol is related to heart disease, but the theory that eating fat causes high cholesterol which causes heart disease is not straightforward. Instead, eating more fat and less carbohydrate, in the context of an overall healthful, whole foods diet, is a beneficial strategy.

Other things that improve your "cholesterol profile" are:

- Losing weight
- Exercising
- Eating vegetables and other high-fiber foods (e.g., seeds)
- Avoiding fried foods
- Avoiding packaged baked goods

The ketogenic diet alone will get you at least half of the things on this list. The rest is up to you.

Triglycerides

Triglycerides (TG) are another type of fat molecule in your blood that doctors measure when you go for your annual physical exam. Having too much TG in your blood raises your risk of heart disease. (You may also be aware that triglycerides are the storage molecules for fat in your body, and there are many thousands of them in your fat tissue.) Although the simplistic thinking would suggest that eating a lot of fat causes you to have more triglycerides in your blood and fat cells, it turns out that it is not so simple as "fat in food" = "fat in the body" (and if it was, you probably wouldn't be reading this book!).

If eating fat doesn't cause high blood triglycerides, what does? According to the National Heart, Lung, and Blood Institute, the major contributors to high triglycerides are:[10]

- Being overweight
- Lack of physical activity

---

10   From the US National Library of Medicine's health information sheet on triglycerides, available at http://www.nlm.nih.gov/medlineplus/triglycerides.html. Last accessed on September 2, 2014.

- Smoking
- Excessive alcohol use
- A very-high-carbohydrate diet
- Certain diseases and medicines
- Some genetic disorders

If you want to reduce triglycerides and thus reduce your risk of heart disease you must lose weight, exercise, and eat fewer carbohydrates!

The Atherogenic Lipid Triad

No, this isn't the name of a warship in *Star Wars*, but it is just as scary. The Atherogenic Lipid Triad refers to three conditions that greatly increase one's risk of atherosclerosis, often leading to heart attack or stroke. These conditions are described individually above.

To summarize, the following factors are known to increase risk of heart disease:

- High levels of TG
- High levels of small, dense LDL particles
- Low levels of HDL particles

As we have seen, too much carbohydrate exacerbates this scenario, and reduction in carbohydrate tends to improve it. Not surprisingly, this atherogenic lipid triad is typically seen in people with impaired ability to metabolize glucose, such as those with obesity, insulin resistance, metabolic syndrome, and type 2 diabetes.

Fats Found in Foods

Cholesterol and triglycerides in the body are directly related to heart disease risk. I hope that now you have a good sense of how these particles affect health. Now let's take a closer look at the types of fats found in foods and how disease risk can be manipulated by diet.

Saturated Fats

Saturated fats are solid at room temperature. Things like lard, coconut oil, and the fat on the edge of your T-bone steak are mainly saturated fats. Saturated fats are good for cooking foods at high temperatures because they don't break down easily with high heat.

The role that saturated fats play in heart health is still a highly controversial issue in the mainstream medical community. Although saturated fats are not considered the certain evil they once were, the average physician will still tell you to minimize consumption of saturated fat for good health—especially if you have high total cholesterol. This isn't surprising given the decades of medical education that have drilled into the brains of physicians (and everyone else) that high cholesterol is bad for the heart, and that saturated fat causes high cholesterol. Expect this type of thinking from your healthcare provider, and bring along a dose of patience if you encounter one who tries to discourage you from following a high-fat, low-carb diet.

The good news is that the medical community is beginning to accept the "saturated fat is okay" message, and a few years from now, this probably won't be such a hot-button topic. There is a wonderful saying, often attributed to the nineteenth century philosopher, Arthur Schopenhauer, that sums up the current thinking on saturated fat in the nutrition community: "All truth passes through three stages. First, it is ridiculed. Second, it is violently opposed. Third, it is accepted as being self-evident." Consider yourself an early adopter.

That said, do not use the ketogenic diet as an excuse to go on a six-month beef-and-cheese-only binge! The average person who switches to a ketogenic diet will increase their saturated fat intake, in many cases by a good amount, just by starting the diet. **It is not healthful to eat a diet loaded with saturated fat and little else.** Eat a mix of saturated and unsaturated fats from a variety of sources! If you are not in the habit of eating fish, nuts, seeds, avocado, or olive oil, now is the time to start.

Monounsaturated Fats

Monounsaturated fats (MUFAs) are found in high concentrations in olive oil; avocados; nuts, such as almonds and pecans; and seeds, such as pumpkin and sesame seeds. Monounsaturated fats are more fragile than saturated fats and can break down more easily with heat and exposure to air. MUFA-rich oils, like olive oil, are good for using cold (e.g., in salad dressings) or for cooking briefly at lower temperatures (e.g., sautéing) but should not be heated to high temperatures or exposed to air. Keep them tightly sealed in a cool, dark place, and don't plan to keep them for months.

Monounsaturated fats are widely considered an important component of a healthful diet and are encouraged pretty much across the board. Surprisingly, there is very little controversy over this point! Despite differing viewpoints over the influence of other types of fats on human health, you would be hard-pressed to find a knowledgeable healthcare practitioner who doesn't espouse the benefit of monounsaturated fats. The Mediterranean diet, broadly touted as "heart healthy," is considered so precisely because more than half the fat calories in this dietary pattern are in the form of monounsaturated fat (largely from olive oil). A higher intake of MUFAs is consistently linked to a lower risk of heart disease and, in some cases, a lower risk of cancer. Make an effort to include MUFA-rich foods like olive oil, avocado, high-oleic sunflower, or safflower oils daily in your ketogenic diet.

Polyunsaturated Fats

Polyunsaturated fats (PUFAs) are found in high concentrations in certain nuts and seeds and their oils, as well as fatty fish.

Polyunsaturated fats are another area of controversy. These fats are very fragile and break down easily with exposure to heat and air. Because of this, they are also easily oxidized in the body and can cause harmful "free radicals," which damage body cells and speed up disease processes and aging. If your diet contained mostly PUFAs (not recommended), this instability in the fat molecule could become a health concern. This fragility also dictates how PUFAs should be used in food preparation: store these oils in the refrigerator in tightly sealed dark bottles to minimize exposure to air and light, use them for cold preparations such as salad dressings, and do not heat them. Once you notice an "off" smell coming from these oils, sort of a musty scent that may be hard to discern at first but will be quite different from the fresh smell the oil had on first opening, throw it out. This odor signals rancidity, the particular spoilage that occurs when oxygen damages a fat molecule, and, unfortunately, means the fat is no longer good for consumption. (If you find this hard to grasp, just remember that rancid oil is like moldy bread. Would you want to eat that?) Polyunsaturated fats are particularly susceptible to this spoilage (monounsaturated fats are less so, and saturated fats are the least fragile) and, as mentioned, this oxidation can also occur in the body and damage tissue cells, resulting in disease.

Moreover, most oils that are high in polyunsaturated fats, such as soy, corn, safflower, sunflower,[11] and cottonseed (as well as products made with these ingredients) are highly likely to be genetically modified unless they are certified organic.[12] Genetically Modified Organisms (or GMOs) are suspected to cause quite serious and long-term damage to health and should be avoided when possible. If you eat a typical American diet with a lot of processed and prepared foods, chances are that you consume a majority of fats as PUFAs from the oils mentioned above. They are used in everything from breads to dips to breakfast cereals. Following a ketogenic diet will get you off of most processed foods and likely lower your consumption of PUFAs, but you still have the choice of which oils to use in cooking and preparing your own foods. *Do not* fashion your ketogenic diet primarily around polyunsaturated vegetable oils. Instead, *consume* polyunsaturated fats along with monounsatu-

---

11   Safflower and sunflower oils can be highly polyunsaturated or highly monounsaturated, depending on the variety. Look for the term "high-oleic," which tells you the oil is at least 70 percent monounsaturated.

12   USDA tracks the percentage of genetically engineered crops. Nationwide in 2013, 90 percent of the corn crop, 90 percent of the cotton crop, and 93 percent of the soybean crop was genetically engineered. Organic certification prohibits the use of GMOs. If you can't find organic, look for the "Non-GMO Project Verified" logo.

rated and saturated fats as part of a mixed-fat diet. (Have you noticed a theme?)

Tip: Unsaturated Fats Are Highly Perishable

It is important to understand that unsaturated fats spoil easily. Unlike shelf-stable foods like all-purpose flour, pasta, or cane sugar, which can last months or even years in your cabinet, unsaturated fats will spoil quickly with exposure to air, heat, or light. Store these in the refrigerator or in a cool, dark cabinet and use them quickly. Don't store fats near your oven or other heat-generating source like a water heater or hot pipes. If you have cooking oil that's been gathering dust and grease above your stovetop for months, chances are it's rancid. Smell it so that you know how to identify rancidity the next time around, and then throw it out.

The Essential Fatty Acids

The category of polyunsaturated fats contains within it another category of fats called the *essential fatty acids*: omega-3 and omega-6 fats. It's essential to consume these because the body cannot make them on its own.

Omega-3 Fats

Omega-3 fats are widely encouraged because they have beneficial effects in the body and because most of us don't get enough of them in our diet. There are three omega-3 fats of interest:

- **Alpha-linolenic acid (ALA)** is found in high amounts in chia seeds, ground flaxseed (and flax oil), walnuts, and canola oil, and in small amounts in some green vegetables, such as Brussels sprouts, kale, spinach, and salad greens.

- **Eicosapentaenoic acid (EPA)** and **docosahexaenoic acid (DHA)** are found mainly in fatty fish, such as salmon, mackerel, sardines, anchovies, and herring; sea vegetables such as seaweed and algae; and in smaller amounts in the meats and eggs of land animals whose diets are rich in omega-3s (some wild game roam on pasture that provides a good amount, and some farmed animals are fed diets fortified with omega-3s—you may see the term "DHA-fortified" on some cartons of eggs). Alpha-linolenic acid (ALA) is converted in the body to EPA and DHA; however, the conversion rate is rather poor, and so it is wise to consume EPA and DHA directly. Because the food sources of EPA and DHA are limited, many people choose to consume these fats in supplement form (see "Not All Fish Oils Are the Same" on page 54).

Omega-3 fats protect against heart disease by improving cholesterol profiles and lowering triglycerides, and they also help relieve symptoms of many chronic diseases, including arthritis, depression, and dementia. EPA and DHA are the building blocks for hormones that regulate immune function, and DHA in particular is important for cognitive function and brain development, especially in children.

Not All Fish Oils Are the Same

Most people fail to consume the recommended two servings of fish per week, and their intake of omega-3 fats suffers accordingly. Because of this, supplements of fish oil containing omega-3 fats are becoming a popular alternative. There are even prescription fish oil supplements used to lower triglycerides.

Most research on the heart health and anti-inflammatory effects of omega-3s highlights the benefit of EPA and DHA specifically, and not all supplements will contain these in good amounts. Look for a product that lists the amount of EPA and DHA on the label rather than one that just says "omega-3s" or "fish oil." A range of 1–2 g of EPA + DHA is commonly recommended to relieve symptoms of inflammation, and up to 4 g is used to lower triglycerides.

Omega-6 Fats

Omega-6 fats are also essential because our bodies cannot make them. But omega-6 fats are not widely encouraged because we tend to consume too much of them already, and because too much omega-6 can have damaging effects in the body. There are two omega-6 fats of interest:

- **Linoleic acid (LA)** (not to be confused with the omega-3 fat, ALA, discussed above) is found in high amounts in various vegetable oils, including safflower, sunflower, corn, cottonseed, and soybean oils.

- **Arachidonic acid (AA)** is hardly found in foods, but is present in small amount in meats, poultry, and eggs. Linoleic acid is converted in the body to AA.

Although omega-3 and omega-6 have similar names, they produce very different effects in the body. In general, omega-3 fats *lessen* inflammation, while omega-6 fats *promote* inflammation. This is one reason why omega-3s are effective in relieving symptoms of chronic inflammatory diseases.

The ratio of omega-3 to omega-6 matters more than the total amount consumed. The average American consumes a lot of omega-6 (from the soybean, corn, and other vegetable oils used in most processed foods) and way too little omega-3. Many experts agree that the ideal ratio of omega-6 to omega-3 is 1:1, but the typical American diet provides at least *ten times more* omega-6 than omega-3! That's a ratio of 10:1—much too heavy on the omega-6 side (and some estimates put the ratio even higher, at 25:1). If you're in the habit of eating packaged foods, the focus on fresh foods in the ketogenic diet will likely reduce your intake of omega-6 fats. It is also a good idea to increase your intake of omega-3 fats. A good way to get omega-3 fats is by eating fish two or three times a week, or by including the omega-3–rich chia seeds and flaxseeds in your regular diet. Omega-3 or fish oil supplements are another common source.

Artificial Trans Fats

Artificial trans fats are created in food manufacturing for use in processed foods so that they can sit on the shelf a long time without going bad. These fats are prevalent in things like crackers, cookies, pastries, chips, and other snack foods, as well as margarine, French fries, and other fried foods. Artificial trans fats are quite dangerous, and they should not be consumed in any amount. They trigger inflammation and are implicated in heart disease, stroke, diabetes, and insulin resistance. Research shows that for every extra 2 percent of calories from these fats daily, the risk of heart disease increases by 23 percent.[13] (Interestingly, naturally occurring trans fats, present in small amounts in meat and dairy products, do not appear to cause these negative effects.)

Artificial trans fats are so dangerous that many cities have banned their use in restaurants. In 2013 the FDA began putting in place measures to effectively remove them from the food supply. But for now, they are still around. So how do you find—and avoid—them? Food manufacturers are required to list the amount of artificial trans fat in their products on the Nutrition Facts panel. However, if an item contains less than 0.5 g per serving, the label can legally read "0 g trans fat." Instead look at the ingredient list: if you see the term *partially hydrogenated oil* then the item contains artificial trans fat.

The good news is that you will be eating little to none of the foods that typically contain artificial trans fats on your ketogenic diet, and so you won't have trouble avoiding them!

---

13   The Nutrition Source, "Fats and Cholesterol: Out with the Bad, In with the Good," Harvard School of Public Health, available at http://www.hsph.harvard.edu/nutritionsource/fats-full-story. Last accessed on September 2, 2014.

Nutritional Benefits and Key Characteristics of Recommended Fat-Containing Foods

Avocado. The avocado might just be the king of the ketogenic diet. The pit in the middle makes it technically a fruit, but unlike other fruits the avocado is full of fat and almost free of digestible carbs. Also, more than 70 percent of the fat in an avocado is of the beneficial monounsaturated type that is widely promoted for good health. Sliced avocado is good on a lot of things, and pureeing it into sauces and dressings gives them a creamy richness. It's even good in smoothies and desserts. You can ripen hard avocados by putting them in a paper bag on the counter for a day or two.

Beef. Although many people think that "beef = saturated fat," beef actually has about equal proportions of saturated and monounsaturated fat. A very small percentage of the fat in beef is of the polyunsaturated type, although the meat of grass-fed animals is a bit higher in omega-3 fats. Grass-fed meat also has more vitamins (especially A and E) and antioxidants, and grass-fed animals are raised in healthier conditions than animals raised in feedlots and fed on grains. Accordingly, the meat of wild game (e.g., deer, elk) tends to be richer in healthful nutrients than standard feedlot meat because these animals eat a variety of plant foods as they roam freely.

Brazil nuts. Brazil nuts are sort of the blank slate of the nut family. They have a very mild flavor, and a lot of vegetarian or vegan recipes will use them ground and seasoned in place of cheese or meat. Try them ground as an alternative to ground almonds in some recipes that call for filler, like meatballs.

Butter. After years of anti-fat diet advice it's hard not to say *yaaaay butter!* Butter tends to make many things way more delicious (eggs and mushrooms come quickly to mind). Butter is about two-thirds saturated fat and one-quarter monounsaturated fat. Grass-fed butter has a higher vitamin content and a richer flavor than typical butter. Make sure to keep your butter sealed in its package or it will pick up flavors from your fridge.

Chia seeds. Chia seeds are crunchy little things that look like poppy seeds. They have an amazing nutritional profile, including 35 percent fiber and the highest proportion of omega-3 fats of any plant food (60 percent of the seed's fat is ALA). The fiber protects the fragile fats in the seed's core, so chia seeds don't spoil easily. Sprinkle the seeds on anything that strikes your fancy, including salads, chicken, yogurt, and smoothies. They add a nice texture with little to no flavor.

Coconut oil. Coconut oil is a major ketogenic diet star. Most of the fat in coconut oil is of the saturated type, but what's special about this source of fat is that 60 percent is in a form called MCTs (or medium chain triglycerides). MCTs are unique in that they are absorbed directly and metabolized immediately in the liver for energy. In contrast, fats that contain "long chain triglycerides" (the majority of fats) must first be broken down, packaged into new forms, and then transported around to other body cells before they can be used for energy. (It is during this voyage that fats may get stuck in the lining of arteries; and since MCTs don't take this trip, they are generally not considered dangerous to heart health.) If you're feeling sluggish on your ketogenic diet, especially in the beginning, the MCTs in coconut oil may be a tremendous help in getting your body the energy it needs. Also, MCTs trigger ketosis, the metabolic state that makes the ketogenic diet so effective for weight loss (the effect of MCTs on ketosis is discussed in greater detail on page 136). Lastly, and perhaps more importantly: coconut oil is just delicious. Use it well!

Flaxseeds/flaxseed oil. Flaxseeds, like walnuts, contain a lot of the fragile omega-3s that are healthy but spoil quickly. It is best to buy flaxseeds whole and grind them just before using (a coffee grinder works great for this purpose). If grinding as you go is not practical, buy ground flaxseed in an opaque bag and store in the refrigerator. If you buy flaxseed oil be sure to get one in a dark-colored jar and use it quickly (it goes great in smoothies and on salads).

Olive oil. Fresh olive oil is a staple in any kitchen. There are many different varieties, and you can explore brands to find ones that are more peppery, citrusy, earthy, buttery, etc. Some specialty shops will have olive oils out for tasting, so take advantage of that when you see it (of course, don't eat the bread used for dipping). Olives and their oil have about 75 percent of the beloved monounsaturated fat.

Salmon. Salmon is generally a good source of omega-3 fats, although the proportion of fat types will vary depending on the species of salmon and whether it's wild or farm-raised. Wild salmon tends to be tastier and comes with the added bonus that you don't have to worry about whether the fish is genetically modified or if it was fed antibiotics with its soymeal feed. Fish roaming the ocean freely generally don't have access to prescription drugs or land crops like soybeans!

Sardines. Some people are turned off by sardines because they usually come in a can. First, sardines are *not* the same as anchovies, which also come in a can or jar. Anchovies are the small, skinny slivers of a reddish pink fish that taste very salty. They are sometimes used on pizza and frequently in Caesar salad dressing. Sardines are much bigger than anchovies, about four inches long, have a silvery-gray skin, and have a milder taste that is both fishy and meaty. Canned sardines from Portugal or Spain are easy to find in the grocery store, and one can often contains more than 1 g of EPA + DHA (the beneficial omega-3 fats). If you're not yet a fan of sardines, a Spanish tapas restaurant is a good place to give them a try. Spaniards eat sardines a lot and they know how to make them taste delicious.

Walnuts. Walnuts tend to be less loved than almonds, and one reason is the perception that walnuts are bitter. Actually, a bitter walnut tastes that way because it is rancid. Walnuts have a high percentage of the fragile omega-3 fats that quickly get damaged with exposure to air, heat, and light. If you've only ever had walnuts from a bag off the grocery store shelf in the baking aisle, then you have likely had the unpleasant experience of biting into a sharply bitter walnut. Fresh-tasting walnuts are absolute buttery deliciousness, and it's worth the effort to find a good source! See if your grocery store carries them fresh in bulk, and find out what day they arrive; then, go buy them that day and store them at home in a sealed container, preferably in the refrigerator.

Putting It All Together

Saturated fat had been uniquely blamed for poor heart health until recently, when several major studies on diet and health failed to find an association between dietary saturated fat intake and heart disease. One of the reasons saturated fat was considered so dangerous is that it increases LDL cholesterol levels. But remember, eating a diet full of the most commonly consumed carbohydrates (breads, sweets, refined grains) increases the small, dense LDL particles that are most dangerous. It is not safe to eat a high-saturated-fat, high-carbohydrate diet. The ketogenic diet is a unique case in which carbohydrates are absent and, even if the amount of LDL is high, this type of diet will likely result in more of the larger, safer LDL particles and less of the smaller kind.

Still, it would be a mistake to fashion your ketogenic diet out of mostly saturated (animal) fats. There is great controversy over the role of saturated fats in heart health. Research on populations with high saturated fat intake and low rates of heart disease, like the Masai people of East Africa, may not be applicable to you and me, because the lifestyles of these groups (e.g., type and amount of exercise, stress level, and so on) are likely very different from ours.

Despite controversy in the saturated fat department, there is broad consensus that increasing the amount of unsaturated fats in general is a good idea. These fats lower LDL and raise HDL, lower blood pressure, and reduce the overall risk of heart disease. They also protect against insulin resistance, and decrease risk of diabetes and metabolic syndrome. Increasing the amount of omega-3 fats in particular (those found in walnuts, salmon, and flaxseeds) is beneficial.

A High-Fat, Low-Carb Weight-Loss Success
Interview with Jimmy Moore

How did you come to be an advocate for the ketogenic diet?

I weighed 410 pounds when I stated the Atkins diet on January 1, 2004. It was my New Year's resolution to lose weight. I was on medications for high cholesterol, high blood pressure, and to help my breathing. My mother-in-law gave me *Dr. Atkins' New Diet Revolution* for Christmas. She'd given me diet books every year, and none had stuck. But I had never tried the Atkins diet, and I was surprised that it said to eat fat and reduce carbs. Every diet I'd ever tried was predicated on cutting fat, cutting calories, and exercising until I was miserable. The reason I failed on those diets was that I was constantly hungry. I was always thinking about when my next meal would be. So I gave this a go. I started on the low-carb, high-fat, ketogenic diet, and lost 30 pounds in the first month. In the second month I had so much energy that I started exercising, and by the end of one hundred days I had lost 100 pounds and I thought, hmm, there's something to this ketogenic thing. In the first year I did go through a period of transition where I didn't lose any weight for about 10 weeks, but during this time I did lose 6 inches off my waist when not a change happened on the scale—and this propelled me to want to do this for the rest of my life. I thought, "This is a sustainable way to eat and a healthy way to eat." By the end of the year I had lost 180 pounds. My personal story is inspiring, sure, but for me, being able to do what I do now—sharing the benefits of the ketogenic diet and helping people—is what matters most.

Why do you think the term "ketogenic diet" is so rarely used?

There's been such a stigma applied to ketosis. It all comes down to ketosis and DKA (diabetic ketoacidosis, a life-threatening condition that occurs typically in uncontrolled diabetics), and the two are not even close to being the same. As long as there is confusion between these terms there will be criticism of ketogenic diets. But now there's a shift toward talking positively about low-carb diets. I've never backed away from using the terms "low-carb," ketogenic, and "high-fat." You look at the latest issue of *Time Magazine*, "Ending the War on Fat," and it's evident. I'm seeing this more and more, people starting to step out more confidently and talk about the fact that carbs used to replace fat in the diet have made people sick. We're going to see some major changes in the way people eat, and a shift from carbs to higher fat, in the coming years.

Jimmy Moore is the author of a number of books, including Keto-Clarity, Cholesterol Clarity, and 21 Life Lessons from Livin' La Vida Low-Carb. His blog and podcast Livin' La Vida Low-Carb are an invaluable resource for the low-carb dieter. Find him at www.livinlavidalowcarb.com.

Key Points

- A high-carbohydrate diet is in many cases *worse* than a high-fat diet for heart health.

- Cholesterol eaten directly from foods has less of an effect on blood cholesterol than the types and amounts of fat eaten.

- There are different types of fats found in different types of foods. Each has unique roles in the body and impacts on health. In general: **Saturated fats** from animal products and polyunsaturated fats from soybean, corn, and other oils found largely in processed foods, should not be eaten in excess; **Monounsaturated fats** such as those in olive oil and avocado, and omega-3 fats such as those in fatty fish, walnuts, and flaxseeds, are encouraged for optimal health.

- A poorly constructed high-fat, low-carb diet can have negative health consequences. Make sure to eat a mix of fats from plants and animals, saturated and unsaturated, for optimal health.

CHAPTER 4

Metabolism for the Ketogenic Dieter

This chapter explains how metabolism works on a carb-heavy diet and on a ketogenic diet. The difference between these is *key* to understanding why the ketogenic diet is so effective for fat loss! And whether you're a science buff or not, learning a bit about metabolism will help you make even better keto food choices to maximize your weight loss.

The Ketogenic Diet at Work

On the ketogenic diet, *most of your calories come from fat*, not protein, as some falsely believe. When you start on a ketogenic diet, you will be consuming about 70–75 percent of calories in the form of fat, 15–25 percent from protein, and the rest from carbohydrate. You will eat between 25–50 g of carbs—at *most* 200 calories' worth—per day. This amount is widely acknowledged as the ketogenic range, although some sources recommend starting the diet at an even lower range (about 12–20 g) to kick-start weight loss. Depending on your individual metabolism and the amount you exercise, you may be able to get away with eating relatively more carbs, or you may have to eat less, to enter and maintain ketosis. You will learn what works for your unique metabolism after a short time on the diet.

Once you've turned on ketosis, you keep it on by *continually restricting carbs*. This is not an 80/20 kind of diet, where you are "good" during the week and "cheat" on the weekends. This is a method of rapid and continual fat loss caused by a shift in the way the body produces energy. Not all low-carb diets accomplish this shift, nor do moments of low-carb eating in an otherwise carb-heavy diet. The shift kicks in when carb intake drops to around 50 g per day or less and stays there. Whether you personally can achieve ketosis consuming 60 g of carbs per day or have to restrict your intake to 15 g per day, one thing is certain: you won't be adding rice to your dinner plate or having a bowl of cereal for breakfast—not even once a week. The small amount of carbohydrate in the ketogenic diet comes from vegetables, nuts, and some dairy foods. If you eat too many carbs you will break the threshold for ketosis and switch back to a carb-dependent metabolism—*and you will stop your diet in its tracks*.

If you truly *want* to stop ketosis, as you may choose to do when you've reached your goal weight, you will slowly and deliberately add carbs back into your diet. You will likely find, though, that once you experience the perks of the ketogenic diet—weight maintenance, stable mood, freedom from food cravings—that you may want to keep your carb intake very low over the long term to continue to reap the benefits.

Since carbohydrates are so important to the ketogenic diet, let's explore the different types and their effect on metabolism.

Are All Carbohydrates the Same?

Carbohydrates are found in food in three basic forms:

1. Starch
2. Sugar
3. Fiber

Starch and sugar may seem different, but they are ultimately the same in terms of how they act in the body. For example, foods like potatoes and rice certainly do not look and taste the same as sweets like soda and ice cream, but they become the same once you eat them. The body converts these foods to glucose within fifteen to thirty minutes of eating them. Glucose is what we are referring to when we talk about "blood sugar," and it is used for energy by every cell in the body. Or, if we eat carbs when the body doesn't need energy, glucose is stored as fat.[14]

Fiber is something different altogether. Starch and sugar are *digestible carbohydrates*, meaning we can break them down to extract energy and nutrients for the body. But we humans don't have the machinery needed to break down fiber and absorb its nutrients. Instead, fiber passes through the intestines, picking up waste products along the way until it's excreted. Fiber is an important dietary component—it's what gives bulk to stools and promotes "easy elimination"—but it does not provide energy (i.e., calories) to the

---

14   The major exception to this rule is fructose, a sugar found mostly in sweet-ened foods and fruit, which is not converted to glucose but rather is converted directly to fat after ingestion. For this reason, some theories suggest that consuming a lot of fructose from things like sugary drinks and packaged desserts may cause rapid fat gain. Fortunately, the ketogenic diet will keep you away from glucose and fructose!

body. This is why fiber is termed an *indigestible carbohydrate*. Most of the fiber in your diet will come in foods that also contain digestible carbohydrate, such as nutrient-rich vegetables, nuts, and seeds.

Starchy and sweet foods like potatoes, rice, flour, corn, apples, bananas, sugar, honey, bread, oatmeal, chocolate, etc., contain a lot of digestible carbohydrates and can easily max out the carb allotment in your diet. Fiber- and water-rich foods like spinach, asparagus, tomatoes, cucumbers, cauliflower, mushrooms, and strawberries also contain carbohydrates, but in much smaller amounts. And, since fiber never enters the body, you can deduct the fiber portion of the food from its carb content to get what we call "digestible" or "net" carbs, which will be a lower number than total carbs. Obviously the more fiber a food has, the lower the net carbs, and thus the lower the contribution to your carb count.

Tip

Think of the ketogenic diet as minimizing *digestible* carbohydrates—starch and sugar.

See the chart "Some Common Foods and Their Carbohydrate Content," on the next page for the fiber and "net" (digestible) carbohydrate content of some common foods from the USDA National Nutrient Database for Standard Reference, version 26. Serving sizes are standard servings or commonly eaten amounts. Carbohydrate amounts are rounded to the nearest gram (g). Note: Do not be fooled by terms such as "Light" or "No Sugar Added" on food labels. These do not indicate that an item is low-carb.

Some Common Foods and Their Carbohydrate Content

FOOD	AMOUNT	TOTAL CARBS (g)	FIBER (g) (indigestible)	NET CARBS (g) (digestible)
GRAINS				
Brown rice	1 cup, cooked	46 g	3 g	43 g
White rice	1 cup, cooked	53 g	<1 g	52 g
Pasta	1 cup, cooked	43 g	2 g	41 g
Oats	1 cup, cooked	28 g	4 g	24 g
Packaged whole wheat bread	1 slice	14 g	2 g	12 g
Homemade whole wheat bread	1 slice	24 g	3 g	21 g
Whole wheat pita	1 medium	20 g	3 g	17 g
Corn tortilla	1 small	11 g	2 g	9 g
Flour tortilla	1 large	24 g	1 g	23 g
FRUIT				
Apple	1 medium	25 g	4 g	21 g
Banana	1 medium	31 g	3 g	28 g
Grapes	1 cup	27 g	1 g	26 g
Strawberries	1 cup	11 g	3 g	8 g
Fresh-squeezed orange juice	1 cup	26 g	<1 g	26 g
DAIRY				
Whole milk	1 cup	12 g	0 g	12 g
Skim milk	1 cup	12 g	0 g	12 g
Heavy cream	2 tablespoons	0 g	0 g	0 g

Cheddar cheese	2 ounces	<1 g	0 g	<1 g
Swiss cheese	2 ounces	3 g	0 g	3 g
Parmesan cheese	2 ounces, grated	2 g	0 g	2 g
Cottage cheese	1 cup	7 g	0 g	7 g
Plain whole milk yogurt	8 ounces	11 g	0 g	11 g
Plain low-fat yogurt	8 ounces	16 g	0 g	16 g
Nonfat fruit yogurt	8 ounces	43 g	0 g	43 g
MEAT, POULTRY, & FISH				
Chicken breast	1 breast, with skin	0 g	0 g	0 g
Chicken leg	1 drumstick, with skin	0 g	0 g	0 g
Beef steak	1 tenderloin	0 g	0 g	0 g
Beef hamburger	3 ounces	0 g	0 g	0 g
Pork	1 chop	0 g	0 g	0 g
Bacon	3 slices	0 g	0 g	0 g
Salmon	3 ounces	0 g	0 g	0 g
Tuna	3 ounces	0 g	0 g	0 g
Shrimp	3 ounces (15 shrimp)	1 g	0 g	1 g
Clams	3 ounces (10 clams)	5 g	0 g	5 g
NON-STARCHY VEGETABLES				
Romaine lettuce	2 cups, raw	3 g	2 g	1 g
Kale	2 cups, raw	12 g	5 g	7 g
Asparagus	1 cup, cooked	7 g	3 g	4 g
Cauliflower	1 cup, cooked	5 g	3 g	2 g

Tomatoes	1 medium, raw	5 g	2 g	3 g
Mushrooms	1 cup, sautéed	4 g	2 g	2 g
Onions	1 cup, sautéed	7 g	2 g	5 g
Jicama	1 cup, raw	11 g	6 g	5 g
STARCHY VEGETABLES				
Potatoes	1 cup, boiled	31 g	3 g	28 g
Sweet potatoes	1 cup, baked	41 g	6 g	35 g
Butternut squash	1 cup, baked	22 g	7 g	15 g
Corn	1 ear, boiled	22 g	3 g	19 g
Lima beans	1 cup, cooked	40 g	9 g	31 g
Green peas	1 cup, cooked	25 g	9 g	16 g
SWEETS & DESSERTS				
Vanilla ice cream (full-fat)	1 cup	31 g	<1 g	30 g
Vanilla ice cream (fat-free)	1 cup	40 g	1 g	39 g
Vanilla ice cream (light, no sugar added)	1 cup	29 g	0 g	29 g
Candy bar—chocolate-covered with peanuts and caramel	1 regular-size bar	35 g	1 g	34 g
Yellow cake with chocolate frosting	1 slice	35 g	1 g	34 g

Remember, throughout this book, the terms "carbohydrate" or "carbs" should be taken to mean net (or digestible) carbohydrates.

Your Changing Metabolism

What is metabolism, anyway? We can say that it's everything that happens in the body—all of the chemical reactions that occur—to convert food into energy. A broader definition says that metabolism is "all of the processes that occur within a living organism in order to maintain life." Wow! Obviously, metabolism is pretty important. Without it, we wouldn't be alive.

Some form of metabolism is happening in our bodies all the time. These processes are *dynamic*, or changing, rather than static and stuck. They will start, stop, or shift to meet varying needs at any given moment. This is fantastic news for someone who wants to lose weight! By taking advantage of your flexible metabolism you can control how your body uses and stores energy.

Basal Metabolism

Most of the energy the body uses on a daily basis goes toward what we call *basal metabolism*. This is the energy the body requires to keep the heart beating and blood circulating, to maintain body temperature, to breathe in and out, and to transmit hormonal and nerve signals throughout the body. You may have heard of "basal metabolic rate," or BMR, which is the rate at which your body consumes energy for these purposes. BMR varies with age, height and weight, and body composition. As a reference point, the average person who needs 2,000 calories a day uses 1,200–1,400 of them for basal metabolism.[15] The remaining 600–800 calories are used for everything else a person does if they're not just laying motionless in a bed: moving around, picking things up, exercising, solving problems, laughing, etc.

If the body experiences a period of starvation or calorie-restriction, as may occur with dieting, it will conserve energy by lowering its basal metabolic rate. When this happens, a person needs to expend more energy (e.g., exercise more) for a given number of calories eaten to avoid gaining weight. This is one reason why someone on a low-calorie diet may plateau after a few weeks of weight loss.

It turns out that the reduction in BMR accompanying weight loss is strongly influenced by the macronutrient composition of the diet.[16] High-fat, low-carb diets appear to *prevent* the reduction in BMR, so these dieters continue to burn more energy for basic body functions as weight loss progresses. This is a considerable advantage of the ketogenic diet that allows for easier long-term weight loss.

---

15   The Harris-Benedict Equation is most often used for calculating Basal Energy Expenditure (BEE). The formulas are as follows: Women: BEE = {655 + (9.6 x wt in kg) + (1.8 x ht in cm) - (4.7 x age in yr)}, Men: BEE = {66.5 + (13.8 x wt in kg) + (5 x ht in cm) - (6.8 x age in yr)}.

16   Ebbeling, C. B., Swain, J. F., Feldman, H. A., et al. "Effects of Dietary Composition on Energy Expenditure During Weight-Loss Maintenance." *JAMA* 307, no. 24(2012): 2627–2634.

Energy for the Body

There are five types of molecules that provide energy to the human body. These are also called "macronutrients."[17] Three of these—carbs, fats, and protein—we know of as important to human nutrition. Two others, ketones and alcohol, are seldom referred to as "macronutrients," but they, too, provide energy to the body. Some of these molecules have other important roles in addition to providing energy.

What Is a Calorie?

You probably know that we measure energy from food in units called "calories." A calorie is actually a unit of *heat* (heat is a form of energy). This is why we talk about "burning" calories when we are fueling the body in exercise.

One calorie is defined as the amount of heat needed to raise 1 g of water 1°C. (This is actually a very small amount, and the energy in food is really measured in "kilocalories," equal to 1,000 calories and abbreviated as *kcal*, but it is common practice to use the word "calorie" instead. For all intents and purposes, unless you are conducting laboratory research, the terms "calorie," "cal," "kilocalorie," and "kcal" are equivalent, and are referring to the kilocalorie).

---

17   Micronutrients—the vitamins and minerals—are equally important to human nutrition. Micronutrients are distinct from macronutrients in that they don't provide energy and are needed in smaller amounts, but they are still essential to human survival.

Carbohydrates provide four calories of energy per gram. Once ingested, carbohydrates are broken down to glucose and used (or stored) in the body exclusively for energy. Carbs are not part of any structural element like bones or eyeballs, nor are they part of any functional molecule like enzymes or hormones (and it's bad news if they are found attached to these molecules, which is something that occurs in people with chronically high blood sugar). Unlike the macronutrients protein and fat, digestible carbohydrates are not nutritionally "essential" for humans.[18] That is, you don't need to eat them. Your body will make all the glucose it needs without any help from your sweet tooth.

Proteins provide four calories of energy per gram, although the body avoids using proteins for energy because they have so many other important functions. Muscles, organs, bones, and skin are made of protein. The enzymes that catalyze the reactions in our body are 90 percent protein. Antibodies, the important immune system responders that fight infection, are proteins. Some hormones, like insulin, are also proteins (recall from page 53 that some hormones are fats). Some proteins, like hemoglobin and albumin, carry things around our blood (in this case, iron and fatty acids, respectively). Because proteins are essential to so many body systems, the body prioritizes using proteins to replenish this machinery rather than breaking them down for energy. So long as we eat enough calories to meet our needs, proteins will be "spared" for these other functions. Failing to consume protein in the diet has severe conse-

---

18   Some carbohydrate foods also contain other nutrients that are essential, such as the vitamin E found in wheat germ or the vitamin C in oranges. Luckily, these essential vitamins are found in many different foods, including keto-friendly foods like sunflower seeds, almonds, broccoli, and Brussels sprouts.

quences, including decreased resistance to disease, muscle wasting, and eventually, death.

Fats provide nine calories of energy per gram. Fats are used in the body for energy and have other important functions as well. Most of us know that fats are stored in fat cells, but few know that fats are found all over the body as well. After fat tissue (or "adipose" tissue), the second highest concentration of fats is in the brain and nervous system. Fats are a physical support for neurons and their connections in the brain, and they make a protective covering for nerves throughout the body. Fats surround the vital organs to protect them from damage while we move around. They are a necessary structural component in cell membranes, forming a wall through which nutrients and waste pass. Fats are also a part of the sex hormones testosterone and estrogen, and the important—but often misunderstood—compound cholesterol. There are many types of fats with varying functions, and the body can make some that it needs from other types—but it cannot produce all that it needs without a dietary source. In other words, fat must be consumed in the diet. Without it, a person will develop deficiency disease and eventually die from malnutrition.

Ketones provide four-and-a-half calories of energy per gram. Like carbs, ketones are not a required dietary nutrient and the body can make all the ketones it needs without a food source. In fact, ketones don't come from food at all. Instead, they are made out of fat in the body. Ketones provide only a small amount of energy when carbs are being consumed and step up to provide a lot of energy, mostly to the brain and central nervous system, when carbs are restricted.

Alcohol provides seven calories per gram. Many people fail to account for the energy provided by alcohol in their diet; thus it contributes to their weight gain. Alcohol, as you probably know, has no essential function in the human body. It is exclusively a source of energy, and too much of it can cause a number of problems, including vitamin deficiencies, excess weight, liver damage, and eventually, death.

Glucose Comes from Three Sources

Glucose is *always* present in the blood, even on a ketogenic diet. *How much* glucose is in the blood depends on what you eat, how much you exercise, how old you are, and how healthy your metabolism is.

There are three ways for glucose to get into the blood:

1. Absorption from the intestine after ingesting carbohydrate. There is very little of this on the ketogenic diet, since carbohydrate intake is kept very low.

2. From the breakdown of glycogen, the storage molecule for glucose. Since glycogen is depleted within the first day or so of carbohydrate restriction, it is not a source of glucose on the ketogenic diet.

3. From the creation of new glucose molecules in the liver, a process known as gluconeogenesis. As mentioned before, the body can manufacture all the glucose it needs from other molecules. The liver constructs glucose out of amino acids (from proteins) and a part of a fat molecule called

"glycerol."[19] Gluconeogenesis is happening all the time, even on a carbohydrate-rich diet. It is the only major source of glucose on the ketogenic diet.

What happens to glucose once it's in the body? If you're eating a carbohydrate-rich diet then your body's cells will be in the habit of using glucose for energy. Your muscles, organs, and brain will pick up glucose from the blood. The hormone insulin plays an important role in this process. (As we will see, on the ketogenic diet, muscles and most other tissues stop taking in glucose for energy and start using fat instead, and the activity of insulin is greatly diminished.) Since your cells are always hungry for glucose on a diet that provides it, they'll also want some sugar in between meals, which they'll get from the breakdown of glycogen in your liver. So when you eat carbohydrates, some of it is also used to replenish glycogen stores. Finally, any excess carbohydrate you consume above what your body needs for energy will be turned into fat and stored in your fat cells. Remember, your body can turn some molecules into others—and it can turn carbohydrates into fat. If you eat too many carbs, that's exactly what happens.

Measuring Blood Sugar

Blood glucose or blood sugar is measured in "milligrams per deciliter" (mg/dL). This describes the *concentration* of sugar in the blood. It's sort of like when you mix flavored powder with water to make a drink like iced tea or lemonade. The more powder you put into the water, the more concentrated the drink becomes. Just as your drink tastes sweeter when

---

19   For this reason, it is important to eat sufficient protein on the ketogenic diet to provide the liver with amino acids for glucose production, thus avoiding the breakdown of important body proteins for this purpose.

you add more powder, your blood is sweeter with a higher concentration of glucose—and this is *not* good!

A normal range of blood glucose is 70–100 mg/dL, and somewhat lower for an individual on a ketogenic diet. Glucose levels *higher* than normal indicate insulin resistance or diabetes, and thus an inability to properly metabolize carbohydrate. The body of a healthy person maintains the appropriate level of blood glucose very well through hormonal activity over the short term, regardless of diet. Over the long term, excessive carbohydrate consumption will lead to insulin resistance for a good many people. For this reason, the ketogenic diet (and low-carbohydrate diets in general) can help prevent insulin resistance and diabetes.

Glycogen

Glycogen is a chain of glucose molecules stored in the liver and skeletal muscle. It's there to fuel the body between meals when it's operating on a glucose-based metabolism.

A dip in blood glucose causes the liver to break down glycogen and send out glucose molecules one at a time into the bloodstream. Unlike fat stores, which hold over 130,000 kcal—theoretically enough energy to last for months—glycogen holds only 1,600 kcal and is depleted in about a day. When all the glycogen has been depleted, the body turns to its fat cells as an energy source and, as long as you don't eat carbs, ketosis sets in.

A person on a fat-based or keto-adapted metabolism does not require glycogen, and, accordingly, has none. Instead, a keto dieter continually makes glucose out of amino acids and glycerol in gluconeogenesis (gluco = glucose, neo = new, genesis = create).

People Need Sugar Like Dogs Need Oranges

For centuries, sailors who spent long periods at sea would develop a disease that caused bleeding gums, painful bruises all over the body, and likely, death. It was believed that a combination of a lack of fresh foods and the stress of being at sea contributed to this disease, although it was unknown why. It was eventually discovered that oranges and lemons cured the condition. Of course we now know that vitamin C in the citrus fruits is what cured the sailors of scurvy.

Vitamin C, like other vitamins and minerals, certain amino acids, and omega-3 fats, is essential to the human diet. But not all mammals require a food source of vitamin C. Dogs and cats, for example, can produce their own vitamin C. Humans lack some of the enzymes needed to make this nutrient. So, we say that vitamin C is an *essential nutrient*—for humans, but not for dogs!

The Institute for Functional Medicine, a respected education and research organization for healthcare practitioners, has a useful acronym for remembering the essential nutrients:

POMFAB

- Protein
- Oils (Fats)
- Minerals
- Fat-Soluble Vitamins
- Antioxidants
- B Vitamins/Methylation Factors

Carbohydrates are conspicuously absent from the list. Carbohydrates appear to be non-essential to humans. This is undoubtedly a controversial point in the realm of nutritional science, in part because of the seemingly "radical" language (i.e., we have for so long considered carbohydrates a *necessary* part of a healthy diet that it's odd to come out and say plainly that we just don't need them). Yet from a metabolic perspective this idea holds true. There is no known disease of glucose "deficiency" that occurs when carbohydrates are not consumed, and humans can manufacture all the glucose we require— just like dogs can make their own vitamin C.

Where Do Proteins Fit In?

Proteins are used for myriad body functions and structures, as described earlier. In a person eating sufficient calories, very little protein is broken down for energy. However, on a ketogenic or very-low-carb diet, proteins are used to produce glucose in gluconeogenesis. For this reason, eating too much protein can interfere with ketosis. This point is an important one because many people believe that the ketogenic diet is a high-protein diet and that consuming huge amounts of protein will increase muscle mass. The ketogenic diet is a high-fat diet, *not* a high-protein diet! And while it's true that the body needs *sufficient* protein to create new muscle tissue, eating more than you need won't magically build up your biceps. It's exercise—*not* overeating—that makes your muscles grow bigger. In fact, the only thing that will grow if you eat too much protein (or anything else) is your fat deposits! Just like excess calories from carbs, if you take in more energy than you need in the form of protein, your body will happily turn it into fat for storage.

Fat Storage and Use Is Controlled by Hormones

Most of the fat in our bodies and in the food we eat is in the form of *triglycerides*. Triglycerides (TG) have three fatty acids attached to a glycerol molecule. When we eat, TG must be broken down into these four parts to pass through the intestinal wall. Similarly, stored fat must be broken down before it can leave fat tissue. The fatty acid portion is used to fuel body cells directly, and the glycerol is used to make glucose in gluconeogenesis. The more fatty acids there are in the bloodstream, the greater the percentage of the body's energy needs they will meet. So if we want to lose fat mass, it is in our interest to enhance the release of fatty acids from fat cells.

This process of *lipolysis* is controlled by numerous hormones in an extraordinarily complex system that is well beyond the scope of this book. However, it will be helpful to understand the basic actions of two important hormones on fat cells. What follows is a very simple explanation of the roles of *insulin* and *glucagon* in fat metabolism.

Insulin Prevents Fat Breakdown

Insulin is released when carbohydrates (and to a lesser extent, proteins) are consumed. Insulin has many actions, one of which is to prevent lipolysis. Insulin blocks the action of hormones that break down triglycerides in the fat cell and allow the fatty acids into the blood to be used up by other cells for energy.

When insulin is low, as after an overnight fast, the fatty acids are released from fat cells and their concentration in the blood is high. When insulin is high, as after a carbohydrate-containing meal, the release of fats from storage is slowed or stopped.[20] In short, when insulin is around, our fat cells stay fat. When insulin goes away, fats come out to play. Indeed, one of our aims with the ketogenic diet is to maintain consistently low insulin levels so that fats may be released from storage and readily used for energy.

Insulin Promotes Fat Storage

Insulin also promotes lipogenesis, or the creation of new fat molecules for storage. Insulin is an *anabolic* hormone; that is, it helps create or "build up" new tissue, including fat cells and proteins, from available nutrients. Insulin does this in part by stimulating cells to take up glucose. Muscle cells that take up glucose use it for energy. When insulin prompts fat cells to take up glucose, they use it to make glycerol, the backbone of triglycerides. Fat cells normally take up glucose and fatty acids simultaneously, and thus have the building blocks for triglycerides. Therefore, storage of triglycerides after a meal is dependent upon the amount of glucose and insulin present in the blood.

Glucagon Promotes Fat Breakdown

Glucagon is a *catabolic* hormone, meaning it breaks down rather than builds up body tissue. Glucagon generally pro-

20   It is problematic to have an excess of both fatty acids and glucose in the blood. This situation can lead to insulin resistance. This is one reason why a high-fat, high-carb diet is not recommended.

duces the opposite effects of insulin. Glucagon levels increase as blood glucose drops, and it prompts the release of glucose from glycogen, release of fatty acids from stored triglycerides, and stimulation of gluconeogenesis. In short, glucagon helps the body use up energy. Consumption of carbohydrates rapidly increases insulin and reduces glucagon levels, returning the body to a state of fat and energy storage.

Is Insulin the Villain?

Let's be clear: insulin is an important hormone, especially if you are eating a carbohydrate-rich diet. People who cannot make insulin, like those with type 1 diabetes, would quickly die without insulin injections. In addition to moving glucose into body cells and preventing fat from getting out of them, insulin has other "anabolic" or building-up effects—one of which is the building up of body proteins. For this reason it has been suggested that individuals on a ketogenic diet may struggle to build new muscle tissue while losing fat; however, studies of keto-adapted athletes have shown that this isn't actually a problem after all. As with many scientific questions, the controversy continues. What we know for sure is that it is important to eat sufficient protein on the ketogenic (or any) diet, both for the body's functional needs as well as to prevent the breakdown of too much muscle protein for gluconeogenesis.

What is important to know is that if your goal is fat loss, too much insulin in your blood can seriously undermine your efforts. You want to minimize the amount of insulin released into your bloodstream so that you can maximize the use of fats for energy. And one of the keys to the ketogenic diet is that by eliminating carbohydrates you minimize the presence of insulin.

Turning Fat to Sugar

We commonly hear that sugar can be turned into fat, but fat can't be turned into sugar. This explanation helps people understand that extra calories from carbs (and any other macronutrient) will be stored as fat. But biochemically speaking, fat *can* be turned into sugar; specifically, the glycerol part of a triglyceride molecule is paired with amino acids (the units of a protein molecule) to make new glucose molecules in gluconeogenesis. The amount of glycerol used in this process varies because it is also possible for new glucose to be made exclusively from amino acids. How much glycerol is used depends on how much extra fat you're carrying and how long you've been off carbs. The more fat you have to lose, the more of it will be used for gluconeogenesis.[21]

Ketosis: Getting the Brain to Run on Fat

Now that we understand how the body gets energy from the three calorie-containing macronutrients—fats, protein, and carbs—let's take a closer look at what happens when we restrict carbs and why this causes rapid fat loss.

Ketones are produced in the liver when fats are broken down for energy. This is happening all the time, regardless of diet. But the liver only produces a small amount of ketones if glucose is around, and, in that case, ketones provide just

21   Paoli, Antonio. "Ketogenic Diet for Obesity: Friend or Foe?" *International Journal of Environmental Research and Public Health* 11, no. 2 (2014): 2092–2107.

a *teeny bit* of energy to the body. However, if there is little or no glucose to be found, the liver grabs a bunch of fat molecules, ramps up production of ketones, and voilà, you have entered ketosis! In ketosis the body may use ten to twenty times the amount of fat-derived ketones as it does on a carb-rich diet!

A lot of these ketones are destined for the brain. The majority of cells in the body can easily use fats for energy when glucose is not around, but the brain *cannot* use fats. When you eat carbs, your brain gets all of its energy from glucose: about 120 g of glucose, or 480 calories' worth, per day. When you don't eat carbs, the brain still gets a little bit of glucose from gluconeogenesis (remember, that's the production of glucose in the body from fat and protein), but nowhere near enough to power all of the important things the brain needs to do each day—like transmit signals through the nervous system to move your arms and legs, or remind you that it's your mom's birthday, or help you understand this book.

Just like a hybrid engine needs gasoline to keep the car driving when the battery runs low, the brain needs an alternate fuel to keep it going when glucose is low. So what does the brain turn to in its time of need? *Ketones.* And what are ketones made from? *Fat.*

When you take away carbs you transform your brain, an organ that uses almost 500 calories of energy per day and which normally does NOT use fat, into a fat-burning machine. On a carb-rich diet the brain will use glucose for 100 percent of its energy needs. On a ketogenic diet the brain will use ketones made of fat for one-half to three-quarters of its energy needs. That's 250–400 calories per day that was provided by glucose that's now provided by fat—and without

you even lifting a finger! If that's not a convenient strategy
for getting rid of fat, I don't know what is!

To Have the Metabolism of a Bird

Even though we may not be thrilled about our love
handles, we should pay them some gratitude. Our fat
stores allow us to go for long periods without eating.
That means we can get a lot of other things done in a
day, and we can even survive for weeks with no food
in an emergency (although it's not recommended). In
a way, this is a nice reprieve; it gives us a break from
having to find and eat food all the time.

Some animals are not so lucky. Take the hummingbird:
the little bird has the fastest metabolism of any animal
alive. It's so fast, in fact, that they must eat all day long
just to stay alive. The tiny animal's heart may beat up to
1,200 times per minute and flap its wings up to eighty
beats per second. In order to have enough energy for
all this, hummingbirds must *always* be looking for
food, and can spare only brief moments of rest between
meals. Each day, the animal must eat 1.5 to 3 times its
weight in food! The little creatures live their lives just a
few hours away from starvation.

Can you imagine being forced to eat all day long just to
stay alive? It sure gives you a different perspective on
dieting!

You might be thinking: That *is* pretty cool…but why doesn't
the body just make more glucose? If you remember from
a few pages ago that "the body can make all the glucose
it needs," you could ask why the switch to ketones occurs
at all. Since the liver is already making some glucose on

the ketogenic diet, why doesn't it just make as much as the brain needs and skip this ketone business altogether?

The problem with making unlimited amounts of glucose inside the body is that both fat and protein are required to do it. The body can't "spare" much protein for energy because it is needed for other essential body functions, like carrying oxygen around the body, metabolizing nutrients, detoxifying waste products, fighting infection, and just about every other important thing the body does. Oh, and let's not forget that unlike fat, of which we have a large supply in storage, there really is no storage form of protein. If your body is forced to use protein for energy it will take some away from your muscles (and not just your biceps, but also more vital muscles, like your heart) and from the pool of proteins performing the tasks named above. Things start to go downhill pretty fast when the body turns to protein for energy—a person would become weak and listless, vulnerable to disease, and, in a short time, would die. This is the fate of a body experiencing starvation.

Instead of allowing itself to come quickly to this dismal end, the body uses ketosis as a "metabolic loophole" to spare protein. The brain's ability to use ketones—*derived solely from fat*—as a major fuel rather than relying on glucose produced from fat *and* protein is really the body's strategy for surviving starvation. Because of this metabolic trick, a normal-weight, healthy adult could survive 30 days of starvation, and an obese person can survive even longer. (See table below for an overview of the body's fuel stores.)

Ketone Chemistry

Here is a quick look at some ketone chemistry:

There are three major ketones: acetoacetate and D-3-beta-hydroxybutyrate provide the majority of ketone calories, and a third ketone, propanone, is used in small amounts.

For someone who IS NOT on a ketogenic diet:

- Ketone levels in the blood will be very low, typically less than 0.3 mmol/L (ketones are measured in "millimoles per liter").

- Ketone levels will be highest in the morning, after the person has awoken from an overnight "fast." The level will drop quickly once they eat breakfast.

For someone who IS on a ketogenic diet:

- Ketosis sets in when ketone levels reach 0.5 mmol/L or greater.

- A ketone level anywhere from 0.5–5 mmol/L is considered normal.

Some references consider ketones levels up to 7–10 mmol/L to be acceptable for a ketogenic dieter. However, higher levels can cause the blood to become overly acidic (a condition called "acidosis"), which is very dangerous. A person with a metabolic disorder, such as diabetes, has a high risk of developing acidosis and may run blood ketone levels as high as 25 mmol/L if they were to attempt a ketogenic diet. For this reason, the diet is NOT recommended for someone with a metabolic disorder except under strict medical supervision. A person with a healthy metabolism who follows a ketogenic diet will most likely maintain ketone levels in the normal range.

Estimates of the Body's Fuel Stores

FUEL	AMOUNT IN TYPICAL 145 lbs PERSON	ENERGY	LENGTH OF ENERGY SUPPLY (if only energy source)
CARBOHYDRATE			
Free glucose	12 g	48 kcal	30 minutes
Glycogen	450 g	1800 kcal	18 hours
Fat (as triglyceride)	15 kg	135,000 kcal	55 days
Protein*	12.5 kg	50,000 kcal	21 days

These numbers are estimates only.

From: Frayn, Keith N. Metabolic Regulation: A Human Perspective. 2nd Edition. Hoboken, NJ: Blackwell Publishing, 2003.

*Body protein cannot all be used for energy because protein is required for necessary life functions, so the body would not last long enough to use the twenty-one days' worth of protein.

Luckily, you *don't* have to starve yourself in order to turn on ketosis! You can just make the body *believe* it's starving by cutting off the glucose supply to the brain, and it will turn ketosis on for you.

Other Tissues Use a Mix of Fuels

Just as the brain can use glucose or ketones, other organs in the body can use a variety of fuels. This is just one more example of the "metabolic flexibility" embedded in our biology—and further evidence that our metabolism is a dynamic process over which we can have some control. Here are some body tissues and the fuels they use:

- **The heart** gets the majority of its energy from fatty acids. The heart will also consume ketones, and, to a lesser degree, glucose. The heart contains no glycogen reserves and thus picks up these nutrients from the bloodstream.

- **Skeletal muscle** uses a mix of fatty acids, ketones, and glucose for fuel. Skeletal muscle also stores a good deal of glucose—about 1,200 kcal, or three-quarters of the body's total reserve—as glycogen. Fatty acids provide 85 percent of the energy needs to skeletal muscle during rest, and glucose, if available, is heavily utilized during bursts of activity.

- **The liver**, the body's major metabolic organ, produces and distributes most of the molecules used for energy by the rest of the body. The liver itself can use fatty acids, amino acids, and glucose for fuel.

- **Red blood cells** are unique in that they exclusively use glucose for energy. On the ketogenic diet this glucose is provided by gluconeogenesis.

- **Adipose (fat) tissue**, it may surprise you to learn, also consumes energy in addition to storing it. Specifically, fat cells need glucose in order to synthesize triglycerides. When glucose is scarce, triglycerides are degraded and the fatty acids are released into the bloodstream to fuel other tissues as described above.

As you can see, the body is adept at using various fuels for energy. The brilliant strategy of the ketogenic diet is that it allows us to take advantage of this flexibility to increase the proportion of fat used for fuel, and thus increase fat loss.

Like carbohydrates, the major purpose of ketones is to provide energy. But, as we saw above, ketones are barely utilized as an energy source unless carbohydrates are removed from the diet. So getting rid of carbs is the key that unlocks the door to using a *lot* of ketones—and therefore a lot of fat. After a week or two on a carb-restricted diet, most cells use fatty acids directly for energy, and the brain and nerve cells use fat indirectly, through ketones.

Another way to look at it is that *ketones eliminate the need to eat carbohydrates*. Since both carbohydrates and ketones serve only to provide the body with energy and have no other structural or functional purpose, we really can choose which energy-providing molecule to use: carbohydrates, which come from the bread and rice and cupcakes you (over)eat, or ketones, which are made out of the fat you gained by eating so many cupcakes. Given the choice, wouldn't you rather use a source of energy made out of your love handles than one made in the bakery?

Eating Too Much of Anything Will Still Cause Weight Gain

By now you understand that ketones are made from fat molecules, and so it's pretty straightforward to see how ketone production can cause fat loss. But let's be clear—you will have a hard time getting rid of fat in a net sense if you consistently eat more than you need. Just because your body has shifted to using fats as its main energy source rather than glucose does not mean that you now have license to gorge on twice your calorie needs and expect all your fat to melt away in a week. When you are in ketosis, your body will use *fat from any source* to fuel itself. That means that it will use the fats it takes out of your cells, *as well as the fats you eat*. Frequent overeating is not a smart strategy for weight loss, even on a ketogenic diet. If you have difficulty responding to your body's hunger and satiety cues (e.g., if you can't tell when you're full) or if you mostly eat for reasons other than hunger, such as to relieve stress or soothe emotions, then you will want to pay particular attention to the tips in Chapter 5 on controlling emotional eating and practicing mindful eating. Fortunately, as you will see in the next section, it is easier to eat with patience and calm on the ketogenic diet as compared to a carb-heavy diet because the ketogenic diet keeps hunger levels low and stable.

How Does a Ketogenic Diet Promote Weight Loss?

In addition to using more fat for energy on a ketogenic diet, there are other proposed mechanisms for how the ketogenic diet speeds up and increases weight loss, including:

Physical effects

Appetite is suppressed.

- through the presence of ketones in the blood;
- through the effect of ketones on appetite control hormones;
- due to consumption of adequate protein, which increases satiety; and

- by avoiding the insulin peaks and dips that occur on a carbohydrate-rich diet, thus stabilizing blood sugar and appetite.

More fat is broken down on the ketogenic diet, and less is created.

- Lipolysis, or the breakdown of fat, is increased on the ketogenic diet because fat becomes the main energy source for the body.
- Lipogenesis, or the synthesis of fats for storage, is promoted by insulin. The default state on the ketogenic diet is a low insulin level and an active use of fat for energy, so lipogenesis is diminished.

People tend to eat fewer calories on the ketogenic diet.

Psychological effects
- Improved mood and greater energy level, and therefore less eating to soothe emotions or fight fatigue.
- The dieter feels rewarded by rapid weight loss and is therefore motivated to stick to the diet.

Practical effects
- Fewer opportunities for eating because of restriction of a common food nutrient (i.e., carbohydrates).
- Removal of "trigger" foods reduces mindless eating.

How Low Is Low Enough?

For many ketogenic dieters the question will come up: how low-carb is low enough? The answer to this question will depend on where you are in your process of weight loss and a bit on your individual metabolism. As we have discussed, a daily carbohydrate intake of about 50 g per day is the *upper threshold* for most people to maintain ketosis.

It's wise to set a lower-carb limit when you begin the diet. Many ketogenic dieters spend the first month at 20 g of carbs per day. This level allows nearly everyone to maintain ketosis and produces rapid weight loss. Also, 30 days at this level will train your taste buds to enjoy non-sweet, non-starchy foods, and it will give you excellent practice monitoring your carb intake—these experiences will set you up for long-term success in low-carb dieting. After some time at 20 g per day, try increasing slightly to 30 g per day. You may find that you continue to lose weight at this level, and if you don't, you can dial back the carbs. You will need to pay careful attention to how your body responds to the amount of carbs you're eating and adjust accordingly. If you keep losing weight, increase your carb intake in small increments, about 5–10 g, as the weeks progress. If weight loss plateaus, you know what to do—cut back down to the level that worked.

Does Low Carb = Ketogenic?

It is important to understand that not all low-carbohydrate diets are ketogenic. The term "low-carbohydrate" may refer to diets that are anywhere from 5–45 percent of calories from carbs, or 20–225 g per day for a standard 2,000-calorie diet. By now you know very well that 20 g of carbs per day is in the ketogenic range, but 225 g *is much too high* to allow for ketosis. Accordingly, look out for foods and dishes labeled "low-carb," as the majority of these will not be referring to the "low" that we are seeking with the ketogenic diet.

Some point to the success of low-carb approaches like the Zone or South Beach Diets, which restrict certain types of carbs and normally don't go low enough to induce ketosis, and ask why it's necessary to go fully ketogenic at all. Low-carbohydrate diets consistently produce greater weight loss than low-fat diets, even if they are not ketogenic. These diets take advantage of the same metabolic strategies, including stabilizing blood sugar, lowering insulin levels, and enhancing the use of fat for energy. *Low carb, non-ketogenic diets are a good strategy for weight loss, but they don't work as quickly or as dramatically as ketogenic diets.* A ketogenic diet drives metabolism deeper in the direction of fat-over-glucose usage for all the reasons explained in this chapter. Ketogenic diets get rid of glycogen and lower blood glucose and insulin levels, and they produce more rapid fat loss. Indeed, some low-carb diet strategies recommend *starting* in a ketogenic phase if you have a lot of extra weight to lose, and *then* becoming more lenient with carbs when your weight goal is achieved. If you choose to use the ketogenic diet for weight loss, you may be able to transition to a higher amount of carbs after you succeed in losing the amount of weight desired.

Key Points

- The body uses mostly carbohydrate (glucose) and fat (fatty acids) for energy, sparing protein for other important functions (except during starvation). Generally speaking, both fatty acids and glucose are being used simultaneously. But we can shift the amounts we use of each by consuming or restricting carbohydrates; the less glucose and insulin in the blood, the more fatty acids the body will use.

- The ketogenic diet minimizes digestible carbohydrates. Avoid starch and sugar. Stick to high-fiber carbohydrate foods such as fresh vegetables and small amounts of berries. Fiber does not count toward your carb intake.

- There is always glucose in your blood whether you are eating carbs or not. On the ketogenic diet almost all of it comes from gluconeogenesis, or the creation of new glucose molecules from protein and fat, rather than from stored glucose or ingested carbohydrate. Certain cells require glucose for energy. The brain continues to consume glucose for part of its energy needs on the ketogenic diet.

- The body is burning the most fat when insulin is low. Lowest insulin levels occur in the absence of carbohydrates. Much less insulin is needed to metabolize nutrients consumed on the ketogenic diet.

CHAPTER **5**

Motivation, Change, and Support

Getting Ready for Change

You're about to change the way you eat. It's important to know *why* you're making this change and what you hope to achieve. When I begin work with a new client I ask: "What are your goals for nutrition counseling?" The usual answers are: "eat better, lose weight, have more energy, be healthier." If this sounds at all like you, you're in the right place!

Aside from the general desire to "lose weight and feel great," everyone has their own unique set of reasons for changing their diet. Getting a clear sense of *your* personal motivators will greatly increase your chance of success. In the nutrition counseling world we use something called the "Transtheoretical Model of Change" (commonly called the "Stages of Change") to hone in on what's driving someone to change and where they are in the process.

We each have individual experiences, thoughts, and feelings that move us from pre-contemplation through to action and maintenance in any life endeavor. Once we've established and maintained a new routine for a while we may cycle back into pre-contemplation, considering yet another new change. There is no starting or stopping place in the stages of change model, and we can enter and exit the cycle at any point.

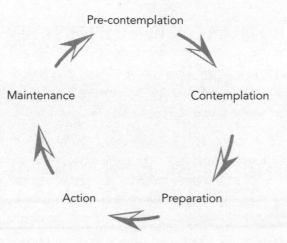

Pre-contemplation

Contemplation

Preparation

Action

Maintenance

For example, let's say one day you decide you want to look for a new job (contemplation). You'll ask yourself if your current job suits your needs and how beneficial it would be to make a change. You'll also consider the difficulties of making a change, as well as the consequences of staying in the same place. Taken together, the answers to these questions will push you or keep you planted. You begin applying for openings (preparation/action) and accept a new position (action). You make the change from the old job to the new one (still action) and stay in your new role for a couple of years (maintenance). After some time you feel a desire to move on (pre-contemplation), but you aren't quite ready to devote real thought to the idea. When you begin thinking seriously of a move, considering what steps you might take to make it happen, that's when you're back in the contemplation phase.

What Motivates YOU? Getting Clear About Your Goals

It's helpful to apply this same process to your decision to change your diet. Identifying your personal, specific motivators and keeping them in mind will help you stay motivated to stick with the diet and maintain your new eating habits over the long term.

So, what motivates *you*? Maybe you've been gaining weight for years and you're finally just tired of it. Maybe you recently had a child and want to be active and healthy for his/her long life. Maybe your doctor recently told you that if you don't lose weight now you'll be on medication for the rest of your life. It doesn't matter what your unique reasons are for doing the ketogenic diet, but it does matter that *you know exactly what is motivating you and keep that in mind* as you move through the phases of the diet.

One of the best ways to increase the likelihood of achieving your goals is to write them down and to have a plan for achieving them. Many of us are familiar with this process in the professional world. In my work with people to achieve their diet and health goals I've observed that those who use this sort of strategy tend to see great results, while those who just "wing it" sometimes do and sometimes don't. You *will* succeed if you plan for success. And as Benjamin Franklin is often quoted as saying: "If you fail to plan, you are planning to fail."

So here is your chance to set yourself up for success. Your needs will change as you move through phases of the diet.

In the very beginning, during the keto transition, you may find that you need more time to sleep, rest, and relax, while a few weeks into the diet you'll likely have more stable energy than you've ever had and you'll be able to exercise easily and be more productive at work. Keeping track of your changing needs and seeking out ways to meet them is essential to being successful at a diet—and it's also a pretty stellar strategy for an enjoyable life! This skill is *resourcefulness*. The fact that you're reading this book already shows that you're resourceful. You knew you wanted to do the ketogenic diet so you bought a guide to help you carry it out. The next step is to do what the book tells you. Ready?

This chapter is about starting out, so we're going to uncover your motivations. Answer the questions below honestly. You don't have to show them to anyone else (unless you want to). This is for you to know why you're doing what you're doing and to help you stay committed to yourself. They'll serve as a reminder as you move through the diet toward your goals.

Worksheet: Why Am I Doing the Ketogenic Diet?

1. What is/are your reason(s) for doing the ketogenic diet? (e.g., *"I want to lose weight," "I want to get rid of sugar cravings,"* etc.)

_____

_____

_____

_____

_____

2. Why are you starting *now*? What's going on in your life that's motivating you now?

_____

_____

_____

_____

_____

3. Describe what your life will be like once you have achieved your ketogenic diet goals. Give as much detail as possible. What will you look like? What will you be doing differently? Paint a picture of the new you. Also, say how you will *feel* once you have accomplished your goals (satisfied, powerful, grateful, etc.).

_____

_____

_____

_____

_____

_____

_____

4a. On a scale of 1–10, how committed are you to this endeavor?

1   2   3   4   5   6   7   8   9   10

4b. If your commitment is less than a 7, list three things
    that would increase your commitment:

_____

_____

_____

_____

_____

4c. Which of the things above are you willing and able to
    do right away?

_____

(*Hint: If you're having trouble, a good way to increase your
commitment to doing the ketogenic diet is to read this
book!*)

Remember, it's *your* decision to do the ketogenic diet, to
lose weight, and to improve your life! You've decided it's
time to achieve *your* goals. Come back to this page anytime you want some self-motivation and a reminder of why
you're doing what you're doing. Keep this around and read
through it often, especially at times when you're contemplating "quitting." If that thought comes up, look at your list
of motivators and ask if any of these things have gone away.
If they're still there, then maybe the action you're taking—
doing the ketogenic diet—is worth continuing.

How Will the Ketogenic Diet Work for You?

Well, what kind of eater are you? Do you cook? Does someone else do your cooking for you, for example a spouse, parent, child, or personal chef? Make sure that person learns the ins and outs of the ketogenic diet as well as you do.

If you're the kind of person who deals easily with change then go ahead and rearrange your kitchen and your grocery list and start eating new foods. If you're the type who needs to have something similar to what you've always had, then you'll need to gather a list of substitute foods to keep you going (check out Chapter 8 "Meal Options" for ideas).

The ketogenic diet is a highly effective strategy for fat loss, and it requires some thoughtfulness to carry out well. You can do an unbalanced version of the KD, eating only bacon and eggs for breakfast, ham and cheese roll-ups for lunch, and a bun-less cheeseburger for dinner—but it's not recommended! *To carry out a healthful ketogenic diet you must eat a mix of animal and vegetable fats, and you must incorporate the non-starchy vegetables that fit into your carb allotment.* Day to day, you must consider how to fill your plate with foods that offer optimal variety and nutrition. Fortunately, this process quickly becomes second nature. As you get familiar with the foods you need on the ketogenic diet you won't have to construct every meal so carefully.

Not everything you eat must have the lowest possible carb content. In the beginning you will want to stick to foods that are carb-free and very low in carbs (e.g., less than 5 g of carbs per serving). Think: meats, fish, cheeses, nuts, avocado, salad greens, oils, unsweetened almond milk, etc. Once you get a handle on the basics of healthy eating and on the amount of carbs in various foods you can begin to allocate your carbs a little more freely. For example, you can have one cup of strawberries, and, knowing that's 8 g of net carbs, you can adjust other meals accordingly.

The bottom line is that you've got to set yourself up to make the diet work for you. If you must have sweet treats every day of your life then you'll want to buy non-nutritive or low-carb sweeteners like erythritol or stevia; you may even carry stevia with you for coffee or tea when out. If cereal with milk in the morning is absolutely a requirement, make a mix of chopped nuts and seeds with some spices and have that with unsweetened almond or flax milk in the morning. Such a mixture is more nutritious and filling than standard breakfast cereal, and just a few bites will make you satisfied—so don't try to eat a whole bowl!

Get the Information You Need at All Times

It's impossible to know the carbohydrate amounts in every food you'll come across, and you may not always know the ingredients in a food—especially when you're eating out. Three things are critical to helping you adhere successfully to the diet.

1. Know how to properly calculate net carbs.

This is largely for packaged foods. The majority of things you come across in packages will have a Nutrition Facts label. To calculate net carbs simply subtract the "Fiber" line from the "Total Carbohydrates" line. That's it. Do not get distracted by the "Sugars" line, as this will just confuse you.

Remember: Net Carbs = Total Carbohydrates – Fiber

2. Carry a food list with you, or download a suitable app.

This is mostly for foods that don't come in packages. The Atkins app is free, and has accurate net carb information for hundreds if not thousands of common foods, as well as different brands of similar foods. It is likely the most trustworthy and relevant app for the ketogenic dieter (recall that the Atkins diet begins as a ketogenic diet and maintains carbohydrate restriction long-term). If a mobile app isn't an option for you, get the booklet version, called "Atkins Carb Counter" (also free), which has the same information and nearly fits in your pocket. (See page 299 for more carb-counting reference sites, apps, books, and other resources.)

3. Ask for the ingredients in anything you didn't make yourself.

This is essential for eating out (or at friends' homes). You mustn't be shy about this! Restaurants make their business by serving you, and when all is said and done, they want the customer to be happy. A busy server may not want to spend extra time tracking down ingredients for you, but, if given the choice, they'd rather do that than have the item returned to the kitchen because it's inedible. *Do not compromise your health or your commitment for anyone*, least of all a total stranger whose job it is to serve you food that's to your satisfaction.

Committing to Your Change

It's widely acknowledged that contracts help people commit to changing their diet and health behaviors. Having someone else *witness* you signing the contract increases commitment even further. It need not be a complicated document (no notary is required!). Simply state in writing that you commit to the ketogenic diet, provide a time frame for your commitment, and sign your name. Ask a trusted friend or loved one to act as your witness. You can use the worksheet below as a sample. Keep your contract in sight as a reminder of your commitment; the kitchen cabinet or your office bulletin board are good places to keep it.

Contract for Commitment to the Ketogenic Diet

Contract

Today's date: _____

I, _____ *[your name], commit to doing the ketogenic diet for _____ [your time commitment, e.g., six weeks, three months]. During this time I will not eat any starch or sugar, except in the small amounts provided by the non-starchy vegetables, nuts, dairy products, and other foods allowed on the ketogenic diet.

Signed: _____
[Your signature]

Witness: _____
[Signature of your witness]

Lining Up Support for Success

Once you've committed yourself to your diet, the last step is to create a hospitable environment for your new lifestyle by asking those around you for support. Think about the things that have helped you through changes in the past, and begin to line up these supports.

Think about your home and work spaces, and your social life. Where do you think you'll find support for your diet changes, and in which places might you run into challenges? Do you live with family, or alone? What are meals like at home? How much real cooking goes on, versus reliance on prepared foods? Do you make time for a real meal during work hours or just get by on the candy and snacks inevitably provided by well-meaning office managers?

I have yet to meet a person, skinny or fat, who tells me they have more than enough time to cook all their meals and who believes that their diet is perfectly healthy, delicious, and satisfying. Dietary perfection is a mirage! We are all operating on a continuum, and the goal is to move, meal by meal, week by week, in a leaner, healthier direction.

You may need some of the people in your life to get on board with your plan. If you live with a spouse or family, it's probably a good idea to let them know what you're doing and educate them a bit about the diet, why you're choosing it, and what you plan to achieve. Then, ask explicitly for their support. Don't assume that people, even loved ones, are able to read your mind and offer the support that you need. *Rather, tell them how they can help you.*

For instance, you might say to your spouse: "It's really important to me to lose weight, and I'm going to do it with the ketogenic diet. I am committed to this plan. I can tell you more about it if you'd like. Right now I want to acknowledge that there will be some challenges, and I am asking for help in advance to make sure I overcome them. Would you be willing to support me in this? It would mean so much to me to have your encouragement. I know I will succeed if I have you on my side."

An opening like this will likely prompt your spouse to promise support and ask what you will need. That's an opportunity for you to be specific. You might say any of the following:

- Would you be willing to keep chips, cookies, and other foods I crave out of the house for a month or two?
- Would you take some time to look at keto recipes with me and try a few in the next couple of weeks?
- Would you say encouraging things when you see me eating a healthy keto meal?
- When we're out with family or friends, would you help me explain why I'm eating this way and encourage them to support me, and especially to defend me if they offer criticism?
- If you see me eating something that doesn't seem to fit on the keto plan, would you find a gentle way to ask me what's going on and steer me back on track?
- Would you refrain from making criticisms about choices that are keto-friendly, and, if you're confused about some part of the diet, would you read the book to learn why the diet is a good move?

Having the support of those closest to you is essential to your success. Ask for these and other things that you need to make it smoothly through this change. Requests like these are perfectly reasonable!

Facing Social Pressure

Your family is a likely source of loving support. They're heavily invested in your life and want to see you be healthy and happy. But others may not be close enough to you to know how best to offer support, so they may say discouraging or insensitive things that can shake your resolve. Worse yet, people who are poorly informed about the ketogenic diet may try to dissuade you from this approach in an attempt to protect your health. It's in your best interest to educate those around you about the diet and its benefits. Be sure to clearly express that you're committed to the diet and excited about this change. Assure them that you have informed yourself and ask them to support your decision. Below are some sound bites to help you through conversations with inquisitive family and friends.

- The ketogenic diet is highly effective for weight loss.
- The diet is high in fat and very low in carbs. It is not a high-protein diet or a meat-based diet.
- I'm eating fat from a mix of plant and animal sources.
- Fats include things like: avocado, olive oil, cheeses, nuts, seeds, and coconut oil. I'll eat these foods along with vegetables like leafy greens, mushrooms, asparagus, tomatoes, cucumbers, and celery, and protein foods like chicken, fish, meat, tofu, and eggs.
- Vegetables are included in the diet, but only non-starchy kinds, like greens, broccoli, and asparagus. No potatoes or corn.

- I'll lose weight faster on this diet because my body will be on a fat-based metabolism instead of a glucose-based metabolism. But in order to do that I have to strictly avoid eating carbs.
- I won't eat carbohydrates like flour, bread, sugar, rice, grains, cereals, potatoes, or fruit.
- Even though there are healthful nutrients in some carbohydrate foods, eating those foods prevents the metabolic change that causes fat loss during the ketogenic diet.
- Our bodies makes "ketones" from the fat stored in cells to fuel the brain when there is no sugar, and that's what gives the ketogenic diet its name.
- Some people are afraid of the ketogenic diet because of a belief that eating fat causes heart disease. This theory has not been proven true. In fact, eating too many carbohydrates is linked to heart disease, obesity, and diabetes.
- The ketogenic diet is also known as a "very-low-carbohydrate" diet. Carb intake must be low enough to promote "ketosis," or the making of ketones from body fat, so just a little "cheating" with carbs is really not worth it.
- I've considered the pros and cons of various weight-loss strategies and have decided that the ketogenic diet is the best one for me. My goal is to lose ____ lbs and enhance my health. It will be easier to do with support from those around me.
- Please support me in sticking to this plan by respecting my food choices and encouraging my success.
- I hope you can offer your support!

CHAPTER **6**

Ketogenic Diet and Health: Taking Care of Yourself

The ketogenic diet is for most people a major change in their way of life. The average person trying to follow standard weight loss advice eats a lot of carbs and steers clear of fat. Now this book is telling you to eat fat, while avoiding carbs like the plague. You'll have to get on board psychologically and emotionally to put these changes into place. As you'll see below, you'll also have to overcome your (likely) negative view of sodium, another food nutrient you have probably made an effort to avoid, because the ketogenic diet increases your need for sodium. This chapter will prepare you for the physical changes that accompany the shift from a glucose- to a fat-based metabolism and guide you in caring for yourself during the transition, as well as through your progression on the ketogenic diet.

Transitioning to a Fat-Fueled State

We talked a lot about ways to successfully manage change in general in Chapter 5. This section will focus on the specific changes that are likely to take place as you transition to a ketogenic diet. Keep in mind that the keto transition does not affect everyone in the same way, although there are some common experiences. Learning how to care for yourself during this time will help keep you going strong.

How Will I Feel?

There is a good chance that you will experience a noticeable lack of energy as you transition to a fat-based metabolism. This period usually lasts about a week, but it can be as short as one or two days, or as long as a few weeks. This could feel like your body is just drained, similar to how you might feel the day before you come down with a cold. You may experience some light-headedness, dizziness, or generalized weakness and just feel like sitting or lying down. Your brain may be "foggy" and it may be a struggle to perform complex mental tasks. You might have a deep fatigue in your muscles and require great effort to lift your limbs. You may have some nausea, diarrhea, constipation, or, in some cases, vomiting. Or you may experience none of these things.

These side effects are, for the most part, normal physiologic responses to the changes occurring in your body. You've likely been on a glucose-based metabolism your whole life. Your brain and body cells know how to work on a fat-based metabolism, but because you have likely never spent days or weeks without carbohydrates, the machinery that works on fat metabolism is a little rusty. This shift is literally straining your body cells all the way down to your DNA. The genes that code for the proteins that help your body metabolize fat have been underutilized. Once you start eating a lot of fat and avoiding carbs, these genes will ramp up to make more and more of the appropriate proteins for the task at hand. But it takes a while to start the gears turning. During that time your body cells have a hard time getting the energy they need. Their main source of food, glucose, is gone, and they don't yet have all the tools they need to feast on the available fats and ketones. It's sort of like landing in a foreign country after a long flight and wanting a nice meal but having only US dollars in your wallet. You have to wait until you find an ATM to get the currency that will let you take advantage of the foods in the new place.

So the keto transition can feel like you lack the energy currency to perform your daily tasks, and in fact, you do. Sometimes you may just need to lay down and rest while your body finds its way in the new environment. There are other things you can do to help minimize the side effects and smooth the transition.

How to Make a Smooth Transition

1. Prepare a calm couple of weeks to start the diet.

If you are exhausted you'll want time to rest and conserve your energy. You won't want to be running around doing errands or going to social events. If you have a demanding job or overly busy family life, see what you can do to create an eye in the storm. Start the diet when you know there will be down time at work, and clear the kids' activity calendar for a couple of weeks. Don't begin the diet when you know you have family coming to town or a big presentation coming up at the office. You may even consider taking a few personal or sick days off from work. The keto transition can feel like an illness, and your mental clarity and physical stamina may be diminished.

2. Drink a lot of fluids.

Ketosis is dehydrating both because glycogen is depleted (glycogen holds water) and because the kidneys excrete more sodium and water during this state. Dehydration can cause headache, dizziness, sleepiness, and constipation— some of the most common symptoms reported during the period of keto transition. It follows that hydrating sufficiently can help prevent or lessen these side effects. Drink *at least* 8–10 cups of water a day, and sip broths and herbal (non-caffeinated) teas as desired.

3. Add salt to your foods.

If you're fearful of salt then you will suffer on the ketogenic diet. The Recommended Dietary Allowance (RDA) for sodium is 1,500 mg/day, but the average American consumes more than twice that amount (3,436 mg/day). That's too much for someone on a carbohydrate-rich diet, but not for someone on a ketogenic diet. Ketosis increases your body's requirement for sodium, and too little of it can cause tiredness, disorientation, headache, muscle cramps, and nausea. By some estimates, a ketogenic dieter requires an additional 2–3 grams of sodium per day.

Get in the habit of adding salt to your foods and drinking sodium-rich broths. You will have a particularly increased need to replace sodium if you spend some hours sweating from exercise or in the hot sun. Remember that water and sodium go together, and one of the reasons your body loses water during ketosis is that your kidneys are getting rid of salt. Put another way, replacing the salt lost in your urine or through your skin will help you retain water and thus stay hydrated. This will, in turn, prevent a lot of the unpleasant symptoms described above.

Giving the Body What It Needs

Well before I ever even thought of doing the ketogenic diet I had an experience in which my body went through a dramatic physiological change—most noticeably in the flavors I craved in my food. I had always been amusingly obsessed with sweets (amusing because I am a nutritionist), and I didn't care much for salty foods. If I craved a snack it was always cake, cookies, or ice cream, and never something like potato chips or cheese puffs. I didn't use a salt shaker at the dinner table and rarely used salt even on foods that demand it, like French fries.

Then, one year, I decided to train for the New York City Marathon: eighteen weeks of running 4-, 6-, and 10-mile runs in the hot summer sun. I'd never done anything like that, and at first I wasn't sure I *could* do it. I finished my first week of training, exhausted as expected, but still pushing ahead. What I didn't expect were the intense cravings for *salt*. I couldn't get enough of the stuff. I began putting salt not just on things that called for it, but on sweet things, too, like my yogurt and granola in the morning. I started carrying a little camping salt shaker around with me.

Clearly I was losing a lot of salt through sweat during my runs, and in the intense heat of the city summer, I was dehydrated. Even though I had never cared for salty things before, my body knew what it needed, and it hijacked my taste buds. It was like salt had some magical power over me; I couldn't go anywhere without it.

I'm not sure I would have made it through that summer of training if I hadn't remembered a recipe for an unusual drink I'd discovered once while traveling abroad. In a beachside town in Turkey, a place where it's generally hot and sunny, I ordered something called a "churchill." It was club soda, lemon juice, and salt. Salt! Most of us are familiar with a drink made of water or club soda, lemon juice, and sugar, aka lemonade. But this was not a sweet drink. *It was a hydrating drink.* In that town, people lived under the hot sun near the beach and they needed rehydration. And in my summer of marathon training, so did I! I drank at least two churchills a day on running days, and one on my off days. The churchill freed me from my salt slavery.

Here is the recipe I used back then, and again while I was on the ketogenic diet:

Squeeze 1 tablespoon of lemon juice (1 g carb) into a large glass. Add ½ teaspoon of salt. SLOWLY pour in 12 ounces of seltzer, club soda, or sparkling water. Do not add the soda too quickly or it will bubble up and overflow!

This ratio of salt and lemon is a good place to start. If you don't notice the salt at all, add a bit more until you can *just* taste it. (Don't add too much or it will be undrinkable. If that happens, transfer the whole thing to a bigger glass and add more water and lemon.)

Tip

A safe, carb-free electrolyte supplement is ElectroMIX, produced by Alacer Corp, makers of Emergen-C. Most grocery stores will stock this product near the nutrition supplements or in the bottled water aisle. Take up to four packets in water daily.

4. Consume foods rich with electrolytes.

In addition to sodium, magnesium and potassium may be important in helping prevent or relieve the symptoms of keto transition. These minerals are "electrolytes," and they help regulate the amount of water in the body, the contraction of muscles, and perform other important functions. Potassium is present in good amounts in a wide variety of whole, fresh foods, but most people on a typical American diet (one based on processed rather than whole foods) do not consume the recommended 4,700 mg per day of potassium. Luckily, a well-balanced ketogenic diet is centered on nutrient-rich whole foods and should not leave you short on potassium. To be sure you're covered, both during transition and throughout the diet, include potassium-rich keto-friendly foods like avocado, nuts, seeds, fish, meat, dairy, and dark leafy greens in your diet. Leafy green vegetables, nuts, and seeds are also good sources of magnesium (the recommended daily magnesium intake is 420 mg for men and 320 mg for women), and meat, fish, and dairy also provide a small amount. On top of food sources, a multivitamin that contains both minerals is a smart addition. Finally, you may add a stand-alone magnesium supplement (no more than 350 mg/day) if you experience muscle cramps, as magnesium helps relieve these contractions. Potassium supplements, on the other hand, are strongly discouraged; excess potassium intake can cause abnormal heart rhythms and may be life-threatening.

5. Sleep as much as you need to.

Unless you are a member of the lucky minority who sails through the keto transition without a dip on your energy meter, you will probably be tired during this time. What do most of us do when we're tired? Have a cup of coffee, a snack, focus even harder on the task in front of us, etc. In our relentlessly busy adult lives we rarely do what any animal would do when it's tired: sleep. So now is your chance to give your body what it needs. If you're dead tired and can't think of anything but your warm bed, act as though you are sick with the flu (which some say the keto transition can feel like at its worst) and go take a nap. Go to bed at 7 p.m. if you need to, and awake when you're rested. If you need to return for another nap a few hours later, do so. You will be bursting with energy once you get into keto metabolism.

6. Eat when you are hungry.

You will likely be very hungry in the first day or two when you're weaning off carbs. If you choose to begin your diet with a fast then you won't be eating during this time. When you finish your fast, or in days three and after, be sure to eat when you are hungry! The ketogenic diet is *not* a starvation diet and you *do not* need to restrict calories or skip meals. It's certainly tempting to try to speed up weight loss by eating next to nothing—especially when you begin the diet and motivation is high. But if you don't eat then you will break down muscle mass and other body proteins for energy, which can exacerbate weakness, increase susceptibility to infection, and make it harder for you to transition overall. Take special care to nourish yourself properly, *especially* in the vulnerable first phase of your diet when you haven't yet gotten into the full swing of ketosis and you may be feeling sluggish. Eat fat, protein, and fibrous low-carb vegetables. Keep appropriate foods and snacks around, and prepare some meals in advance (as you may not want to cook if you are feeling ill).

7. Avoid exercise in the very beginning if you are fatigued.

There's no point in beating around the bush: in your first week on the ketogenic diet your arms and legs may feel like lead. You will try with great effort to climb stairs or lift yourself out of bed, and the possibility of more strenuous exercise will be laughable. (Hopefully you *will* laugh, because you know that this means you're on your way to the fat-burning, energy-enhanced state of ketosis!) *If this is you*, do not exercise during this week. If you drag yourself to the gym you will just be discouraged that you can barely lift half your normal weight or eke out a few minutes on the treadmill before feeling like you've walked forty days and forty nights through a hot desert. You'll crawl home and get into bed, which is where you should have been in the first place! Just remember that you'll feel better in a week or two and you can go back to your exercise regimen or start one. For now, take care of yourself. (If you're not fatigued and exercise comes easily, soldier on!)

8. Avoid alcohol and be smart about your caffeine use.

This is pretty self-explanatory. Alcohol is disorienting and dehydrating, not to mention disruptive to nutrient metabolism. Moreover, a "hangover" can feel a lot like the worst symptoms of the keto transition. No point in making this harder on yourself! Be smart and stay off alcohol for the time being.

Caffeine is a little more complicated. Caffeine is also dehydrating, and if consumed in excess can cause a variety of unpleasant symptoms, including rapid heartbeat, upset stomach, and insomnia. However, *caffeine withdrawal* can bring on symptoms like headache, fatigue or drowsiness, difficulty concentrating, depressed mood or irritability, and even flu-like symptoms such as nausea or muscle pain! Some of these are among the worst things dieters experience in the keto transition. You certainly don't want to add insult to injury by quitting caffeine cold turkey. If you are a habitual caffeine user it's a good idea to either stick to your normal regimen or start weaning yourself off before you start the diet. (If you've gone off caffeine before with no ill effects, then feel free to go without it.)

Does Caffeine Increase Fat Loss?

Caffeine is widely studied for its potential to promote weight loss. Studies show a higher concentration of fatty acids in the blood after caffeine ingestion, which is a sign that caffeine (like the ketogenic diet) promotes "liberation" of fats from fat cells. (However, it is unclear whether caffeine consumption increases the use of these fats for energy.)

There is also good evidence that caffeine increases the Resting Metabolic Rate (RMR), or the amount of energy the body uses while at rest. This is sometimes also referred to as the "thermogenic effect." Just 100 mg of caffeine—the amount in one cup of coffee—can cause a 3 to 4 percent increase in resting energy expenditure. This is equivalent to burning about 50–75 kcal. The effect is small, but over time it can add up.

Despite these promising mechanisms, studies of the effect of caffeine on weight loss have not had convincing results. People who ingest caffeine do not appear to lose more weight than people who don't have caffeine.

So caffeine may not be a fat-dissolving magic bullet for your metabolism in the way that the ketogenic diet is. But don't underestimate the power of a cup o' joe. The science aside, caffeine is probably most effective at promoting weight loss through its practical use. If having a cup of coffee gives you something to do when you would otherwise have a meal or snack, then the beverage may very well be helping you lose weight.

9. Give yourself a break.

If you're feeling ill, irritable, or having trouble concentrating, then you will probably not be operating at your best. You may not be that productive at work, and you may snap at family and loved ones. Sometimes, you may just need to rest, relax, or be alone. Social situations may not be ideal for the moment. Just give yourself a break and take the space you need to refuel. Order delivery for dinner (make sure it's keto-friendly!) if you can't spare the energy to cook. Get a massage, take a bath, listen to music, go to the movies, etc. Do the things you like to do when you're feeling under the weather.

10. Know that it will pass soon.

The keto transition is just that—a transition. Some people feel sluggish for a day or two and wonder what everyone else is complaining about; others feel really sick, and may even think of quitting. Although you may have to endure a week of moodiness and malaise to get there, if you stick with it you will find that being on "the other side" is very worth it. You won't have to suffer those uncomfortable transition symptoms again (unless of course you decide to quit the diet and start over, and the threat of that should be motivation enough for you to stick with it!). On the ketogenic diet you'll have more energy, you'll be thinking more clearly, your mood will be at its best, you won't be hungry, and you'll be losing weight—fast.

What Happens Next?

Congratulations, you've made it through the transition period and you're officially on the ketogenic diet! If you had any symptoms during the transition, that was likely the worst of it and you should be feeling *much* better now. Still, the strategies that helped you through the transition are good practice for the longer haul, so don't become lazy about your self-care. It's still important to drink plenty of water, get enough rest, eat a variety of nutritious keto foods, and follow the guidelines for healthful eating throughout the book.

Now that your body has shifted to a fat-fueled metabolism, a lot of other changes will take place. The next section covers common concerns about body, weight, and health on the ketogenic diet.

How Do I Know If I'm in Ketosis?

If you follow the diet and properly restrict your carbs, your metabolism will shift to a fat-burning state. As you enter ketosis you will very likely experience the transition period described above. If you experience this and don't "cheat" on your carbs, you can safely assume that you're now burning fat. Other signs that you are in ketosis:

- You're not very hungry.
- You get full easily.
- You're losing weight.
- Your energy level is more stable.
- Your mood is better.

You can also measure the level of ketones in your urine with "ketone urine strips" available at any pharmacy. If the color on the strips is anything other than the lowest level, then you are in ketosis.

How Long Can I Be on the Diet?

There is no prescribed amount of time to do the ketogenic diet. It's generally accepted that two to three weeks is needed to induce a good level of ketosis, but if you have a lot of weight to lose you'll certainly want to spend more time on the diet. Weight-loss studies commonly keep participants on the diet for anywhere from a few weeks to many months, and recommend a period of six months to one year to achieve significant weight loss. The ketogenic diet is used in hospital settings for one to three years for treatment of epilepsy. Some professional researchers whose work focuses on ketone metabolism have written books and articles describing a lifetime on the ketogenic diet.

In general, though, the average person using the ketogenic diet for weight loss will follow it for a few months to achieve their weight goal and transition to a more lenient low-carb eating pattern for long-term weight maintenance.

Losing Weight

You will likely lose a few pounds in your first one to two weeks on the diet. This is mainly due to loss of glycogen and water and is not exactly cause for celebration, but it should feel pretty good nonetheless!

After this, the weight you lose will be fat and muscle. Your goal is to minimize muscle loss and maximize fat loss, which can be achieved by:

- Eating sufficient protein. Protein needs are determined by body weight and activity level. Typically, the protein needs of a sedentary person who does no exercise are estimated at 0.8–1.0 g of protein per kilogram of body weight per day (or g/kg/day). Someone who does light to moderate intensity exercise requires an estimated 1.2–1.7 g/kg/day, and for someone who exercises frequently at very high intensity, estimated protein needs are 1.4 –2.0 g/kg/day. A ketogenic dieter gets a greater percentage of calories from protein than the average person on a carbohydrate-rich diet for whom these standards were likely developed (a high-carbohydrate diet is the standard recommendation), so your protein intake can be higher for the given activity level. Eating *too much* protein is not recommended, though, and you should consider 1.5–2.0 g/kg/day to be the upper limit. (Also recall that eating too much protein can disrupt ketosis.) Studies of the effect of the ketogenic diet on body composition (change in fat and muscle mass) have shown mixed results, with some reporting loss of muscle mass, some reporting maintenance, and a few reporting increased muscle mass.

- Eating sufficient fat. The ketogenic diet is not a starvation diet. It's a technique that allows you to make use of your fat stores without enduring the negative effects of starvation, such as muscle wasting. There is an upper limit to both your carb and protein intake for reasons already discussed. So you must get the bulk of your calories from fat. If you are afraid of fat or want to avoid it, you will not succeed on the ketogenic diet.

Exercise

Think back over the years of your adult life. What were the moments when you gained weight? Did something stressful occur? The loss of a relationship or a job, perhaps, or the death of a loved one? Maybe you moved from a warmer to a colder climate, and the time you'd previously spent outdoors being active was now spent inside, eating warming food during cold winters. Maybe your commute to work lengthened, and you ate an unhealthy, fast food breakfast in the car on the way into the office. Perhaps you had a child, and time devoted to self-care began to be used for the care of another, and exercise fell by the wayside. When I ask my clients to tell me about the moments in their life when they gained the bulk of their weight they almost always describe periods of loneliness, increased family or job responsibilities, and a shift away from "leisure" activities, like group sports, toward seemingly "more important" responsibilities, like fixing things around the house. I often wonder how it comes to pass that fixing a leaky faucet is more important than protecting oneself from weight gain and chronic disease!

Family, career, socializing, hobbies, and other activities that keep one happy in life are undoubtedly important, and I don't mean to suggest that these take a backseat! But neither should your health. People often tell say they don't have time to exercise. But if you devote just a little time to caring in this way for your body you will find that you reap benefits in so many areas of your life, including enjoying time with your family in a healthy body for many years to come. Diet can take you a long way toward your weight goals, *but exercise is an essential component of weight loss and maintenance success.* There are many reasons for this, but two points in particular should interest you:

1. The more muscle mass you have, the more energy you use. This is often referred to as "faster metabolism" or "higher metabolic rate." Your body is mainly made up of muscle and fat, along with some bone. The bone mass changes very little over the course of your adult life. Muscle and fat can come and go depending on what you do with your body. Muscle cells need more energy than fat cells, so the more muscle you have on you, the faster you will use your energy—which, if you're already on the ketogenic diet, will be coming largely from your fat stores. The amazing thing is that this happens even when you're doing nothing at all. In other words, as you sit here reading (and probably not lifting weights) your muscles are burning through fuel (namely, fat) relatively

quickly in comparison to the other parts. So, in general, a muscular person can stay thinner than a non-muscular person eating the same amount of calories. The extra muscle on their body is what helps them stay thin. So grow some muscles and let them work for you! In order to get more muscle, you have to exercise.

2. You can eat more carbs if you exercise. Exercise makes your body use up glucose more quickly, so you can eat more carbs and still be in ketosis. Exercise also improves insulin regulation, which, if it's abnormal, will tell your body cells to hold on to stored fat (and make more of it). Luckily, exercise—both aerobic and strength training—improves this situation.

If you're already exercising, keep it up! If you're not exercising, a good question to ponder is the following: what percentage of time per week do you *reasonably* think you can devote to exercise? One percent? Five percent? Let's take a conservative estimate of 3 percent. Three percent of your life devoted to strengthening your body, increasing your muscle mass, "speeding up" your metabolism, and "burning" through your fat stores, not to mention clearing your mind and improving your mood and overall health. Do you think you devote just 3 percent of your time to the cause?

Now tell me: how many hours per week do you exercise? If you said less than five hours, you are spending less than 3 percent of your time exercising.

The Dietary Guidelines for Americans call for thirty minutes of moderate-intensity physical activity (above one's usual daily activity) on most days of the week to reduce risk of chronic diseases like heart disease and diabetes; sixty minutes of moderate-to-vigorous activity on most days of the week to prevent adult weight gain; and ninety minutes of moderate-to-vigorous activity daily to maintain weight loss in adulthood! This is not a prescription that you must follow exactly. You could, for example, do a two-hour intense training session one day and no training the next. There are more sophisticated approaches to exercise, such as interval training, that can reduce the overall time needed for comparable results. However you do it, you must find some time for adequate exercise.

If you think you absolutely cannot find time to exercise, I want you to do the following activity. Make a chart with the days of the week across the top, and the activities you do most often along the side. For one full week, chart the activities that use up your time. Start with the thing that takes up the most hours, which for most people will be either sleep or work. Subsequent entries will be:

- Commuting
- Eating
- Watching TV
- Taking care of kids/family members
- Shopping for and preparing food
- Bathing/personal care
- Exercising
- Hobbies
- Household chores
- Relaxing
- Learning new things/studying
- Socializing

At the end of the week, add up the number of hours you've spent in each activity. Look for two hours that are spent doing something non-essential (hint: household chores and watching TV are usually good places to look), and devote those two hours to exercise. If you can shoot for three, four, or even five hours, go for it! Make your exercise hours part of a feasible, routine activity schedule. For example, you can do four thirty-minute segments Monday through Thursday if you know that on those days you come home in the evenings, whereas on Fridays you usually go out with friends. If weekdays are too booked, consider two one-hour segments on the weekends. Figure out what works for you, and commit to it. Remember, if you increase your frequency and intensity of exercise you will very likely be able to eat more carbs and still maintain ketosis. If you've been sticking to a range of 20–30 g of carbs per day and would like to bump up your daily allotment (to, say, 50 g per day) without stalling your weight loss, exercise is the ticket. So get moving!

Why Am I in a Great Mood?

Feeling great on this diet? I may be the ketones. Ketogenic diets promote the production of gamma aminobutyric acid (GABA), a neurotransmitter (brain chemical) associated with mood disorders. A lack of GABA is linked with depression, mania, and other disturbances. Drugs that promote the production of GABA (called GABA "agonists") are effective antidepressants. They're also used to treat bipolar and manic disorders. More research is needed to determine the effectiveness of dietary therapies for these conditions, and the ketogenic diet is not promoted as a "cure" for depression or mood disturbances. But if your mood is better than it's been in a long time, it may very well be the ketones!

Supplements

There is a world of controversy about the use of supplements for health in general, and the need—or lack thereof—of supplements for health on the ketogenic diet. Health professionals tend to have two major concerns in this regard (and it's important to understand these points because the question of supplements will come up a lot while you're on the ketogenic diet, and in things you read about it):

1. It's difficult to determine supplement quality/ efficacy, because the supplement industry is poorly regulated; and

2. Every "body" is individual, and each person responds differently to changing diet, environment, stress level, and so forth. Blanket recommendations for supplementation may enhance health for some, while potentially harming others.

For this reason, good physicians and healthcare providers will not be quick to recommend supplements based on reports of symptoms, but rather will thoroughly test biomarkers in the blood to assess cellular and organ functioning before they prescribe a supplement. Like any other aspect of health, each person is unique—and each person needs to take an active role in their own care. If you are not feeling well, it's important to find a healthcare provider who will listen to your account of symptoms and assess your overall case, rather than just prescribe blanket treatments.

In addition, the optimal way to get the nutrients you need is to consume them directly from food. As mentioned in the discussion on electrolytes on page 118, some supplements, if not taken properly, can be dangerous.

With those caveats in mind, there are a couple of other supplements that may be useful to the ketogenic dieter. First, as mentioned above, a good-quality multivitamin is a wise choice. When you begin to restrict foods you may miss out on nutrients that were supplied by the broader range of foods in your previous diet. Especially when you first change your diet and you are figuring out what to eat, you may not eat the healthiest, most robust variety of foods. It's impossible to know how you, personally, will fashion your ketogenic diet (although hopefully you will create a healthful diet full of various fats, high-quality proteins, and nutrient-rich vegetables). For this reason, a daily multivitamin is recommended to ensure that you get a minimum of a range of micronutrients. Be aware that some vitamins and supplements (even those in capsule form) have added carbohydrate. Make sure to check the label.

A multivitamin will provide a good foundation as you navigate your new eating pattern. In general, the more restrictive and the less varied your diet is, the greater your risk for nutrient deficiency. Your individual physiology will also play a role (some people metabolize nutrients more effectively than others). If you consistently make poor food choices (e.g., eating bacon and eggs for breakfast every single day, a burger without the bun as your standard lunch, and little to no vegetables), then you may run into trouble. If you eat a rich variety of foods, including fish, nuts, meats, dairy, various oils, and avocado, and you make good use of your carb allotment to get a variety of non-starchy vegetables, then you will likely be in good shape nutrition-wise!

You may also consider supplementation with *medium chain triglycerides (MCTs)*. Regardless of your nutrition status, this is one "supplement" that's really a food component that can be a very helpful tool on the ketogenic diet. Medium chain triglycerides are a type of fat that's found in high concentration in coconut and palm oils. These fats are rapidly absorbed and highly ketogenic—meaning they can kickstart or deepen your level of ketosis if you think you're not quite there. Bear in mind that MCTs also have a laxative effect, which can be helpful to counteract constipation, but not so helpful if you end up with diarrhea and abdominal pain, which is a possibility if you consume too much.

If you want to experiment with MCT oil you can use more coconut oil in your meals. There are MCT oil supplements, which are extracts of just these fats alone (about 60 percent of the fat in coconut oil is in MCT form), but they can be harder to find than common nutritional supplements. Among the handful of products out there are KetoForce, from Prototype Nutrition, and Bulletproof MCT oil (a lot of ketogenic dieters are fond of Bulletproof coffee, a coffee drink with MCT oil and grass-fed butter).

Your interest will likely be piqued by a host of other supplements in addition to those mentioned here—especially those products claiming to burn fat and promote weight loss. Again, the quality and efficacy of supplements varies widely, and some are downright unsafe. If you are determined to include supplements in your regimen I strongly recommend that you work with a qualified healthcare provider to determine your individual nutrient needs.

MORE Carbs? Really?

One oddity is this: Believe it or not, there are reports of some people following a ketogenic diet who for some unknown reason stopped losing weight, and the solution was to *add* some carbs back in. Whether this enhanced weight loss was through ketosis or some other mechanism is unclear, but, so the stories go, the dieters began losing weight again. Oh, and the carbs they ate? Half of a grapefruit per day.

What If I'm Not in Ketosis?

First, make sure you know where you're getting your carbs and that you're not eating too much. Are you reading labels on *all* packaged foods? Are you eating out for most of your meals, and if so, have you made sure that sauces are made without sugar or starch, that meatballs and hamburgers are free of breadcrumbs, and that the little white dots in your salad actually *are* flecks of grated Parmesan and not couscous (a tiny grain of wheat flour)? Is someone else doing your cooking for you, and if so, are they following the guidelines? Do some investigation and see if there aren't some hidden carbs sabotaging your diet efforts.

Next, follow the diet. Be honest with yourself about what you're eating and whether you're cheating. Maybe you nibble just a bite of dessert when someone at your table offers it, or you have half a granola bar at work *only* when you're totally stressed. If you're thinking that just a little bit of sweet stuff here and there won't hurt, get clear about doing the diet, and do it.

Third, check for carbs in things you ingest other than food. Many medications are made with carbohydrate ingredients. Syrups are the worst culprits, but pills and tablets may also have carbs. Do you take a daily vitamin? Have you recently been drinking cough syrup for a cold? Check the labels on these items for hidden sources of carbs. If you discover carbohydrates in something you take regularly, see if you can swap brands or product types for something carb-free. The Charlie Foundation (website listed in the resource section) has a list of low-carb and carb-free products that includes medications and body care items.

If you've made sure you're following the diet correctly and you still suspect you're not in ketosis, try a clear liquid fast for three days. This is the approach used in a hospital setting for patients for whom failing to achieve ketosis could mean significant consequences for their health. Accordingly, this approach is *very* effective. If you can't handle a fast, try:

- Eating less protein. Amino acids from protein are used to make glucose in the body, and eating too much can dampen ketosis.

- Adding MCT oil or coconut oil to your meals. As described above, this will enhance ketosis.

- Eating fewer carbs. Everyone's carb threshold is different. You will have to find out what level works to keep you in ketosis. If you feel you're not there, try cutting back for a few days, and then add carbs back in 5–10 g increments and see what happens.

- Exercising. As described above, exercise will help your body use glucose, keep your insulin in check, and overall give you greater "carb" freedom.

What Is the Difference Between Ketosis and Ketoacidosis?

The subject of ketoacidosis is bound to come up during your journey on the ketogenic diet. It's important to know the difference between a safe, normal level of ketosis and an abnormal, potentially life-threatening state of ketoacidosis.

Ketosis (also called physiologic ketosis) is the body's normal response to fasting or sufficiently restricting carbohydrates. People with properly functioning metabolisms who abstain from food for a period of days, or eat less than 25–50 g of carbs per day (depending on their ketogenic threshold), will enter a state of ketosis. The level of ketones in their blood will be much higher than that of someone eating a carbohydrate-rich diet. These ketones will be used to fuel the brain and other body tissues in the absence of glucose. Importantly, the amount of ketones in the blood of a healthy person in ketosis is normal for the carbohydrate-restricted diet they're on, and their body functions properly.

In contrast, *ketoacidosis* is not a normal condition. Ketoacidosis occurs when the level of ketones in the blood is too high. It most commonly affects diabetics (which is why we often hear of diabetic ketoacidosis, or DKA), but ketoacidosis can also occur in severe alcoholics, people with pancreatitis or kidney disease, those taking certain medications, people with undiagnosed metabolic disorders,[22] and others.

---

22   Undiagnosed metabolic disorders are not rare. Consider a classic example: diabetes affects 29.1 million Americans (or 9.3 percent of the population); 8.1 million of them, or 27.8 percent of those affected, are undiagnosed—meaning they don't know they have it. Source: Centers for Disease Control and Prevention, National Diabetes Statistics Report, 2014, available at http://www.cdc.gov/diabetes/pubs/statsreport14/national-diabetes-report-web.pdf, last accessed September 2, 2014.

Ketoacidosis is extremely dangerous and may even be fatal. Symptoms include nausea, abdominal pain, and vomiting, and, if left untreated, can progress to cerebral edema (swelling of the brain), coma, and death. For this reason, anyone who suspects they may have a metabolic disorder, or anyone who is not in good general health, is advised not to attempt a ketogenic diet unless under strict medical supervision.

Constipation

This is a popular topic in the ketogenic diet world. It often happens that new ketogenic dieters become constipated. According to the National Institute of Diabetes and Digestive and Kidney Diseases, constipation is defined as "a condition in which a person has fewer than three bowel movements a week or has bowel movements with stools that are hard, dry, and small, making them painful or difficult to pass." You may also have pain or bloating in your abdomen. It is *not* true that bowel movements must occur every day. Normal bowel movement frequency is from three times a day to three times a week, depending on the person.

Among the major causes of constipation are:

- Diets low in fiber
- Lack of physical activity
- Medications
- Life changes or daily routine changes

You can see why the ketogenic diet might increase the likelihood of constipation, especially at the start. First, ketogenic dieters are at risk for low fiber intake if they avoid vegetables. This is one reason why non-starchy vegetable consumption is encouraged. Second, the ketogenic diet is likely a major life change that will take some getting used to. Third, as you transition to a fat-based metabolism, in the beginning you may be tired and avoid physical activity.

Thankfully, this problem is easy to correct. If you do suffer some constipation in the beginning, these strategies should help you recover:

- Drink sufficient fluids. Aim for 8–10 cups per day.
- Eat more fibrous vegetables, such as leafy greens and broccoli, and high-fiber seeds, such as flax and chia seeds.
- Eat Hass avocados (these promote bowel movements).
- Include medium chain triglyceride (MCT) oil in your diet. You can buy this as a supplement, or increase your consumption of coconut oil, which contains a high proportion of MCTs.
- Exercise (the best time is fifteen to forty-five minutes after a meal, because eating helps stimulate the colon).
- Take a stool softener or mild laxative.

Adverse Effects

The potential for adverse or harmful side effects exists with any diet scheme. The ketogenic diet may increase this possibility due to the significant changes in body chemistry (e.g., change in electrolyte status) that occur with ketosis. According to the guide *Modified Ketogenic Diet Therapy* by Beth Zupec-Kania, RD, CD, and published by the Charlie Foundation for Ketogenic Therapies in 2013, the ketogenic dieter should be able to identify the symptoms of two serious potential adverse effects and be aware of the treatment for each:

1. **Low blood sugar.** A blood sugar level between 50–75 mg/dL is considered normal for someone on the ketogenic diet, while a somewhat higher range (70–100 mg/dL) is normal for a non-ketogenic dieter. Low blood sugar, or "hypoglycemia," can be dangerous.

   The symptoms of low blood sugar include:
   - Shakiness
   - Heart palpitations or rapid pulse
   - Pale skin
   - Sweaty forehead
   - Dizziness

   Blood sugar that falls below normal levels can be corrected immediately by taking 1–2 g of fast-absorbing carbohydrate, such as one tablespoon of juice.

2. **Excess ketosis.** An overproduction of ketones (i.e., a level above that which is considered normal for the ketosis of the ketogenic diet) can be very dangerous and must be treated immediately.

   The symptoms of excessive ketosis include:
   - Nausea
   - Rapid, shallow breathing
   - Facial flushing
   - Vomiting
   - Extreme sleepiness

Note that excessive ketosis refers to the level of ketones *in the blood* rather than in the urine, so a "small" or "moderate" reading on ketone urine strips *does not rule out* the possibility of excessive ketosis. However, if excessive keto-sis *is* present, the rapid change of color on the test strips (indicating a high level of ketones) can help confirm the condition.

In a manner similar to the treatment for low blood sugar, excessive ketosis can be corrected with two tablespoons of juice. If the symptoms persist after twenty minutes, another two tablespoons of juice is recommend, and the individual is advised to seek medical assistance.

CHAPTER 7

What Can I Eat?

If you want to eat a ketogenic diet and lose weight you have to eat <u>real food</u>. Do not be fooled by naysayers who tell you that there is nothing to eat on the ketogenic diet!

Would You Want Your Doctor to Cook You Dinner?

I've talked with some clinicians and researchers who believe that the ketogenic diet is too hard to follow because it lacks variety. I disagree. I think the problem is that these people don't know a lot about food. They are experts in science and medicine, but what does that say about their interest or expertise in cooking, gardening, and the like? There is no requirement for a medical doctor or a nutrition scientist to know how to cook, and it's a well-publicized fact that few medical schools provide even the most basic nutritional education to future physicians. In reality, the average doctor is likely to know as much about food as your high school biology teacher— which is to say, who knows how much that is?

Ask any chef and they'll tell you there is a <u>world of options</u> available to the ketogenic dieter. Many I have met since beginning my journey with the ketogenic diet have been excited to talk with me about creating something I genuinely want to eat. My own diet has become more varied since I started eating this way, partly because I have been exploring new foods. It's easy to get caught in a rut, eating the same foods day in and day out, but it's not very much fun! The ketogenic diet turned my attention toward foods in which I'd never really had an interest (for no good reason other than the fact that I'd lazily made the same familiar meals year after year). For instance, did you know that you can make "rice" out of cauliflower? One cup of cooked cauliflower has 2 g of net carbs. One cup of brown rice has *40 g of net carbs.* That's a lot of starch! Even if I wasn't on a ketogenic diet I don't know why I would want to eat all that. Unless I plan a brisk run afterward it's all going to turn into fat. Now, thanks to my experience on the ketogenic diet, I know a lot of great recipes to replace starchy foods. I've learned you can also make 100 percent keto-friendly mashed "potatoes," salt and pepper "chips," and pizza crust—*out of cauliflower.* (You can find the recipe for Cauliflower Mashed Potatoes" on page 272.)

Another reason that it's important to focus on foods is that the majority of dietary education is focused on *nutrients:* carbs, protein, fat, calories, saturated, unsaturated, grams, micrograms…huh? It's all a bit abstract, and can be somewhat overwhelming to someone who's not trained in nutrition. So consider this an opportunity to put all that information about metabolism to practical use. While counting carbs is essential to the ketogenic dieter, it becomes much easier to do so once you have a solid understanding of foods.

This chapter is devoted to actual foods rather than nutrients—those foods allowed on the ketogenic diet, those you'll want to avoid, and how to take advantage of the great variety of healthful foods available to you.

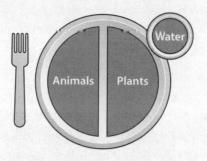

Eating Fresh

One of the things you'll notice on the ketogenic diet is that when you go looking for food you'll be looking in the refrigerator instead of the cabinet. Ketogenic foods tend to be perishable, which is generally considered a positive for nutritional health. Except for nuts, seeds, and oils, which can last for a while at room temperature (although refrigerating them helps to hold off rancidity and is a smart thing to do), as well as some dehydrated vegetable products (e.g., seaweed, kale chips) there aren't many keto-friendly foods that are shelf-stable. It's usually a mix of flour, sugar, and harmful trans fats that allow food products to sit for months on the shelf without going bad (think of powdered doughnuts, breakfast cereal, crackers, and candy of all kinds). Any nutritionist would tell you to eat as little as possible of these foods to avoid gaining weight and becoming diabetic. And yet, most will still criticize the ketogenic diet as unhealthy. It's largely ignorance of the foods eaten on the diet that drives this perspective. If you look closely at the food allowed on the ketogenic diet you'll find that this eating pattern automatically nudges you toward the type of healthful, whole foods diet that is widely recommended for optimal health.

Vegetables

When you hear the word "vegetables" you probably think of things like broccoli and salad greens. You may also think "fat free." Now you're on the ketogenic diet being instructed to eat lots of fat, and here is a list vegetables! You remember from the 1990s that people on the Atkins diet were supposed to stay away from vegetables and stick to meat and animal products. What's the deal?

First, vegetables are importantly separated into starchy and non-starchy types. You will not eat starchy vegetables on the ketogenic diet. Second, it is important to understand that the ketogenic diet is NOT an animal-based diet—and you should be wary of any dietary advice that suggests otherwise. The ketogenic diet includes a mix of animal and plant foods. You must eat vegetables of the non-starchy variety—you must also *count the carbs in them* and be sure you're staying under your threshold of 25–50 g per day, but *you must eat them nonetheless.*

If you're not in the habit of eating vegetables, develop the habit now. Buy a variety of fresh vegetables when you stock up on food for the week, and aim to try new ones as you move ahead with the diet. Frozen vegetables are an acceptable substitute to keep in the house for when you haven't made it to the grocery store.

Now, which vegetables are okay to eat? The following table from the USDA National Nutrient Database for Standard Reference, version 26, gives the carb content of non-starchy vegetables that should be *the bulk of the carbohydrate calories on your ketogenic diet*. Amounts shown are a typical serving size.

All good

Net Carb Content of Selected Non-Starchy Vegetables

DESCRIPTION	AMOUNT*	NET CARBS (G)
Endive, raw	1 cup	0.0
Epazote, raw	1 tablespoon	0.1
Grape leaves, canned	1 leaf	0.1
Watercress, raw	1 cup	0.2
Green onions (tops only), raw	1 tablespoon	0.2
Beet greens, raw	1 cup	0.3
Lettuce (red leaf), raw	1 cup	0.3
Ginger root, raw	1 teaspoon	0.4
Spinach, raw	1 cup	0.4
Arugula, raw	1 cup	0.4
Broccoli raab, cooked	1 cup	0.5
Lettuce (green leaf), raw	1 cup	0.5
Lettuce (romaine), raw	1 cup	0.6
Lettuce (Boston and bibb), raw	1 cup	0.6
Mustard greens, raw	1 cup	0.8
Seaweed (kelp), raw	2 tablespoons	0.9
Seaweed (wakame), raw	2 tablespoons	0.9
Nopales (cactus), raw	1 cup	1.0
Broccoli (Chinese), cooked	1 cup	1.2
Lettuce (iceberg), raw	1 cup	1.2
Turnip greens, cooked	1 cup	1.3
Chinese cabbage, cooked	1 cup	1.3
Shallots, raw	1 tablespoon	1.4
Radicchio, raw	1 cup	1.4
Tomatillos, raw	1 medium	1.4
Celery, raw	1 cup	1.4
Nopales (cactus), cooked	1 cup	1.9

Radishes, raw	1 cup	2.0
Savoy cabbage, raw	1 cup	2.1
Spinach (frozen), cooked	1 cup	2.1
Cauliflower, cooked	1 cup	2.3
Asparagus, raw	1 cup	2.4
Spinach, cooked	1 cup	2.5
Sauerkraut, canned	1 cup	2.6
Garlic, raw	1 tablespoon	2.6
Zucchini (summer squash), raw	1 cup	2.7
Portabella mushrooms, grilled	1 cup	2.7
Green bell peppers, sautéed	1 cup	2.8
Jalapeño peppers, canned	1 cup	3.0
Zucchini (summer squash), cooked	1 cup	3.0
Collards, cooked	1 cup	3.1
Dandelion greens, raw	1 cup	3.2
Cucumber (with peel), raw	1 cup	3.2
Okra, cooked	1 cup	3.2
Cauliflower, raw	1 cup	3.2
Brown mushrooms (Italian or cremini), raw	1 cup	3.2
Hearts of palm, canned	1 cup	3.3
Jalapeño peppers, raw	1 cup	3.4
Kale, raw	1 cup	3.5
Kohlrabi, raw	1 cup	3.5
Mustard greens, cooked	1 cup	3.5
Swiss chard, cooked	1 cup	3.5
Shiitake mushrooms, stir-fried	1 cup	3.6
Broccoli, raw	1 cup	3.6
Chayote, cooked	1 cup	3.6
Fennel, raw	1 cup	3.7
Beet greens, cooked	1 cup	3.7

Savoy cabbage, cooked	1 cup	3.7
Chayote, raw	1 cup	3.8
Asparagus, cooked	1 cup	3.8
Green chile peppers, canned	1 cup	4.0
Tomatoes, raw	1 cup	4.0
Artichokes (globe or French), cooked	1 medium	4.0
Green snap beans, raw	1 cup	4.3
Green bell peppers, raw	1 cup	4.4
Brussels sprouts, raw	1 cup	4.6
Red cabbage, raw	1 cup	4.7
Jicama, raw	1 cup	4.7
Kale, cooked	1 cup	4.7
Turnips, cooked	1 cup	4.8
White mushrooms, cooked	1 cup	4.9
Red bell peppers, sautéed	1 cup	5.1
Yellow onions, sautéed	1 cup	5.3
Green snap beans, cooked	1 cup	5.9
Red bell peppers, raw	1 cup	5.9
Broccoli, cooked	1 cup	6.0
Turnips, raw	1 cup	6.1
Eggplant, cooked	1 cup	6.1
Crushed tomatoes, canned	½ cup	6.5
Peas, boiled	1 cup	6.8
Brussels sprouts, cooked	1 cup	7.1
Spaghetti squash (winter squash), cooked	1 cup	7.8
Leek, cooked	1	8.3

As you can see, vegetables vary in their net carb content. It's important to eat these vegetables on the ketogenic diet, so it's a good idea to know their approximate carb content and choose thoughtfully.

Pesticides and Weight Gain

Certain pesticides are what researchers call "obe-sogenic." These chemicals accumulate in fat tissue and disrupt the hormonal system that regulates fat use and storage, causing people to gain weight. They also cause insulin resistance, which can lead to further weight gain, and diabetes. In addition to the negative metabolic effects, pesticide residues may cause a number of other health problems, including neurological and developmental problems (such as lost IQ points), especially for children.

Buy organic produce whenever possible to minimize exposure to pesticides. You can tell a produce item is organic if it's labeled "organic" or if the PLU code (the number the cashier uses to look up the price) is a five-digit number that starts with a "9" (non-organic PLU codes are four-digit and begin with a "4"). If organic across the board is not an option, use the Shopper's Guide to Pesticides in Produce from the Environmental Working Group (www.ewg.org) to determine which produce items have high levels of pesticide, and at minimum, choose organic versions of those items.

Meat, Poultry, Fish, and Shellfish

Muscle meats from land animals, birds, and fish are carb-free. Shellfish contain a small amount of carbs, as do animal livers and brains.

All Meats

This category includes beef, pork, lamb, bison, venison, goat, rabbit, etc.

When we eat a steak or pork chop we are eating the muscle of the animal. Muscle is made of protein with small fat deposits, and some cuts (like a pork chop) have pure fat around the edges. Feel free to enjoy whole cuts of meat on or off the bone, ground meats, meat broths, and animal fats as you wish.

In particular, meat or bone broths are a great addition to the ketogenic diet. Most broths provide sodium and potassium that are needed in higher amounts on the ketogenic diet, as well as an additional source of fluids. Homemade broths, or those from a butcher shop or farmers' market, tend to be more nutritious. Canned or boxed broths purchased at the grocery store may have unwanted ingredients. Bouillon cubes, powder, or paste almost always contain carbohydrates. Check the labels on packaged products carefully for sources of carbs, and make your own broths or buy fresh versions when possible.

Tip

Tallow (beef fat) or lard (pork fat) are sources of saturated fat that can be used for cooking at high temperatures.

Good Fats from Grass-Fed Cows

It is truly an amazing feat that an animal as big as a cow can be nourished on grass alone—but it's true. If left to their own devices, cows normally eat grass. But in order to fatten the animals for food production, cattle are raised in "feedlots" where they are fed a mix of grains. (If you recall from the writing of Jean Brillat-Savarin, grains make animals—and people—fat!) Although this method produces meat more quickly and cheaply, it is of lower nutritional quality. Grass-fed beef is higher in omega-3 fats, vitamins A and E, and antioxidants. Grass-fed animals are less likely to be given hormones or antibiotics, which are otherwise common in industrial animal production. Look for a label on the product that says "grass-fed" and, whenever possible, purchase this type.

It can be tough to decode the various labels and certifications such as "grass-fed" and "pasture-raised" often used with animal foods. For a quick overview, check out the Environmental Working Group Meat Eater's Guide at www.ewg.org/meateatersguide/decoding-meat-dairy-product-labels.

All Poultry

This category includes chicken, turkey, duck, quail, goose, etc.

If you've been trying to lose weight on a low-fat diet then you've likely been sticking to the skinless-white-meat-only rule with chicken. Well, now is your chance to party! Eat any portion of the meat you like, including the skin.

Like other meats, poultry contains protein and fat, but no carbs.

Antibiotics in Animal Production

Small doses of antibiotics are routinely added to the feed of animals raised industrially for food. These "sub-therapeutic" doses prevent animals raised in close quarters from getting sick—and also causes them to gain more weight than they would without the drugs. It's unclear why this is so, although some theories suggest that the antibiotics kill certain good bacteria in the animals' guts that would help them avoid weight gain. Studies of the differences in gut bacteria of humans who are either overweight or of normal weight suggest that there is a strong relationship between weight status and the type of bacteria in the intestinal tract.

The widespread use of antibiotics in animal production is thought to contribute to the rising prevalence of antibiotic-resistant bacterial infections in humans. These are difficult to treat with current drugs, and healthcare professionals warn that diminished effectiveness of antibiotics may bring about grave consequences for public health.

Stick with meats from animals raised without antibiotics. Certifications like "antibiotic-free" are not formally regulated. To assure that a meat product is antibiotic-free, look for the *organic* label, which prohibits the use of antibiotics. You can also be reasonably assured that no antibiotics were used if you see a combination of one of these claims: "Raised without antibiotics," "No antibiotics," "No antibiotics administered," or something similar, *and* the term "USDA Process Verified," which means that the claim about antibiotic use has been verified by the Department of Agriculture.

Tip

Animals hold glycogen in their muscles and livers just like humans. Muscle glycogen is used up during slaughter, but the liver of the animal will still contain glycogen, and thus a small amount of carbs. The bigger the animal, the more glycogen the liver will contain. If you eat the liver, remember to count the carbs. Popular products are calf's liver, chicken liver, and duck liver ("foie gras").

All Fish

This category includes salmon, mackerel, sardines, tuna, trout, sole, etc.

Fish are a great source of protein and unsaturated fat (including omega-3s), and contain no carbs. Fewer than one in five people eats the recommended two servings per week. Many people are turned off by fish due to fear of mercury contamination. High levels of mercury in fish are indeed a significant health concern; nevertheless, fish are considered such an important component of a nutritious diet that it's worth seeking out high-quality, safe-to-consume varieties. Try these fish that are typically low in mercury:[23]

- Salmon
- Mackerel
- Herring
- Haddock

---

23   For more information on the mercury content of varying fish species, as well as state advisories on contamination of local waterways, see the Natural Resources Defense Council "Consumer Guide to Mercury in Fish," available at www.nrdc.org/health/effects/mercury/guide.asp.

- Trout
- Flounder
- Catfish
- Whitefish

It's easy to find a variety of good-quality canned or jarred fish in an upscale grocery store or specialty foods market. In particular, fatty fish that contain good amounts of healthy omega-3 oils are often available canned. Look for:

- Sardines
- Mackerel
- Salmon
- Anchovies

All Shellfish

This category includes shrimp, scallops, clams, mussels, calamari, etc.

While finfish are carbohydrate-free, crustaceans (like shrimp, crab, and lobster) have a small amount of digestible carbohydrate, and mollusks (like squid, mussels, clams, scallops, oysters, abalone, and octopus) contain a bit more. Enjoy these foods—but count the carbs!

FOOD	NET CARBS (G) IN A 3-OUNCE SERVING
Mussels	6 g
Oysters	5 g
Clams	4 g
Scallops	5 g
Octopus	4 g
Lobster	1 g
Shrimp	1 g
Crab	0.5 g

Source: USDA National Nutrient Database for Standard Reference, version 26

Hidden Carbs in Meat, Poultry, and Fish

Although meat, poultry, and fish are carb-free, some *preparations* of these foods are not keto-friendly. Meat and poultry marinades are often prepared with sugar or honey, and certain cuts of meat are typically sweetened when cooked (for example, ham at holidays). Dried sausages, cured meats, and cold cuts often contain sweeteners and starches used to retain moisture and flavor. You'll want to look at the nutritional facts or the ingredient lists for these items and choose ones without an added source of carbs.

Sauces accompanying fish are less likely to contain carbohydrates than those used with meat or poultry. Whole fish or fillets are commonly prepared with oil, butter, and/or lemon and herbs. Avoid breaded, floured, or fried fish completely. Smoked fish, such as lox or whitefish, may or may not have added sweeteners; check labels. Tuna fish salad is easily made carb-free with some mayonnaise and spices, but it could also contain sugar. Raw fish, as in tuna or salmon tartare, might contain mirin, a sweet rice wine, sugar, and/or other sweeteners. Salmon is sometimes dried into a sort of fish "jerky," usually with a sugary ingredient. Stay away from fish "cakes" or "nuggets" or "sticks," as these are almost always breaded or filled with a starchy ingredient.

Soy Protein (Tofu and Tempeh)

Tofu or bean curd is a mild-flavored food made from mashed soybeans that is popular in vegetarian cuisine. Tofu is low in carbs and is a good food to have on rotation with meat, poultry, and fish as an entrée item. It comes in soft, firm, very firm, and sprouted varieties. The firmer versions can be cooked like any meat item.

Tempeh is a fermented cake made of soybeans that can be low in carbs. It has a nutty, earthy flavor—sort of how you'd expect a bean cake to taste. It's very good baked or grilled if it's been marinated first. Traditional soy tempeh is usually low in carbs, approximately 3 g per 3 oz serving. Other varieties are made from grains, such as rice, and may not be low in carbs. Check the labels.

Dairy Products

Dairy foods are tricky. First, the carb content of dairy products can range from 0 g for heavy cream and certain cheeses, to 45 g per serving for flavored yogurts (most of that coming from added sugar). Second, even low-carbohydrate dairy foods may cause a spike in insulin. If you recall, insulin is a hormone that promotes tissue growth (including fat tissue). Because milk is the primary food of infants, it prompts the release of insulin to help the infant grow. Unfortunately, this is not helpful for an adult seeking weight loss. Dairy foods should be limited to a few ounces per day and carefully chosen to avoid items with added sugar. Still, it's worth the investigation to find keto-friendly products in Dairyland. Use this list as a guide, and look closely at the Nutrition Facts panel to find products with few or no carbs (5 g per serving is a good ceiling).

Good choices are:

- Heavy cream
- Butter
- Cheeses like cheddar, Swiss, brie, goat, blue, feta, etc.
- Tub cheeses like mascarpone and ricotta

- Créme fraîche (fat-free is okay)
- Sour cream
- Fromage blanc
- Cottage cheese
- Plain Greek or Icelandic yogurt
- Quark

Remember, choose *only* unflavored dairy items, and stick mainly to full-fat products. Do not buy any sweetened dairy foods. Reduced fat (i.e., skim, fat-free, nonfat, low-fat, 1 percent, and 2 percent) items often contain sweeteners and starches that are added to replace the creaminess lost when the fat is removed. Be careful when choosing dairy products.

It's a Good Idea to Avoid Hormones in Dairy Products

It is common practice to use growth hormones in dairy cows to increase milk production. You may have heard of recombinant bovine growth hormone (rBGH), also known as recombinant bovine somatotropin (rBST). Milk from cows treated with these drugs has higher levels of Insulin Growth Factor-1 (IGF-1), a hormone naturally found in humans that appears to increase risk of cancer when present in high levels.

These hormones are approved for use in the US but banned in Canada, the European Union, and Japan because of concerns over health risks posed to animals and humans. As with many aspects of food production, this point remains controversial. From a weight loss perspective, it is not hard to see why ingesting hormones in your food is a bad idea: fat use and storage is controlled by a complex hormonal system that, if you're overweight, is already disrupted.

The good news is that it's easy to avoid this potential health risk and weight-loss barrier. Look for the "organic" label, which prohibits the use of hormones, or seek dairy products labeled "hormone-free," "rBGH-free," or "made with milk from cows not treated with rBGH."

Choose Yogurt Carefully

Most yogurts have a significant amount of added sugar and should be avoided by both the ketogenic dieter and anyone who is interested in maintaining a healthy weight. This is especially true of low-fat or nonfat yogurts, but it is also very common in full-fat yogurts. The majority of yogurts will not be suitable for your ketogenic diet. When buying a yogurt, seek high-quality, plain (unflavored) yogurts without additives. The ingredients should be milk and bacterial cultures (some yogurts also contain cream).

Strained yogurts tend to have a lower carb content regardless of their fat content. They have had a lot of the water (whey) portion removed. These are creamy and filling, with a consistency similar to chocolate mousse (you can stand a spoon up in them). Examples are Greek, Icelandic (Skyr), and Turkish or Middle Eastern (lebneh) yogurts.

Instead of yogurt, try:

- **Fromage blanc** is a French cheese that is eaten with a spoon, usually in the morning as a stand-in for yogurt. It has no carbs—not even the fat-free variety—and thus is a great replacement for yogurt if you'd like to avoid the small amount of carbs in that. Add chopped walnuts for an easy breakfast option.
- **Quark** is a German cheese that's very much like a thick yogurt or light cream cheese. Quark typically has fewer

carbs than even a low-carb yogurt. It can be eaten the same way.

Keep in mind that dairy foods—even low- or no-carbohydrate items—promote the release of insulin, which may get in the way of weight loss. Eat these foods sparingly.

Refrigerated Non-Dairy Items

The dairy case is home to a wide variety of keto-friendly items that are not dairy foods at all. Look for these items in your local grocery store:

- Whole eggs
- Liquid eggs
- Tofu
- Packaged sliced meats (without sweeteners)
- Sauerkraut/fermented vegetables
- Kelp or tofu noodles
- Unsweetened nut or seed milks (e.g., almond or hemp milk)
- Guacamole
- Salsa
- Baba ghanoush
- Cheese or cream dips

You'll likely find these and many other acceptable foods in this section. Spend some time reading labels to be sure you're choosing products wisely. Note that some salsas and dips have added sugar, or may include starchy ingredients like pureed beans. Always check labels for net carbs!

Most of the nutrients in an egg—not just cholesterol, but also all of the fat, choline, and vitamin A—are contained in the yolk. Yet it's hard for people who have been trying to follow low-fat diet advice for years to believe that they will not immediately give themselves a heart attack if they swallow an egg yolk. Not so. Your body needs cholesterol to function properly. Cholesterol plays an important role in cell membranes, and it is a building block for the sex hormones testosterone and estrogen. Twenty-five percent of the cholesterol in the body is in the brain, where it's also important for neurological function. Moreover, low cholesterol levels appear to correlate with increased risk of dementia. One egg yolk contains 184 mg of cholesterol. Your body needs about five times that amount, or 1,000 mg of cholesterol per day—and much of that is produced by the body itself!

Fruit

It's best to avoid fruit on the ketogenic diet. A small amount of berries once or twice a week is an acceptable indulgence, but keep in mind that the carbs in fruit add up quickly. Lemons and limes can be used a bit more freely; these are good flavoring agents in meat marinades and dressings, and a squeeze of lemon is nice in seltzer water. Just be sure to count the carbs from these citrus juices.

Carbohydrate Content of Allowed Fruits

FRUIT	AMOUNT	TOTAL CARBS (G)	FIBER (G)	NET CARBS (G)
Lemon juice	2 tablespoons	2	0	2
Lime juice	2 tablespoons	2	0	2
Rhubarb*	1 cup	5	2	4
Blackberries	1 cup	14	8	6
Raspberries	1 cup	15	8	7
Clementines	1 fruit	9	1	8
Cranberries*	1 cup	13	5	8
Asian pear	1 small fruit	13	4	9
Strawberries	1 cup	12	3	9

Source: USDA National Nutrient Database for Standard Reference, version 26

*These fruits are *very* sour and in almost all cases are mixed with sugar to make them palatable; unfortunately, the sweetened versions are not suitable for eating on the ketogenic diet.

Deli Counter and Prepared Foods

The deli counter has a great selection of keto-friendly foods but it can also be a source of hidden carbs. Read the nutritional facts or ingredient list on any item with a label, and ask about the ingredient content of unlabeled foods. The following are good ketogenic diet choices IF they don't contain starches or sweeteners:

- Sliced meats (e.g., proscuitto, roast beef)
- Dry sausages
- Gourmet cheeses
- Tuna, chicken, or egg salad
- Pickled vegetables (e.g., pepperoncini)

Hidden Carb Tip: Look out for sweeteners and fillers in sliced meats and sausages; honey or fruit in gourmet cheeses; sugar in pickled items; and olives stuffed with items that may be high in carbs (such as sundried tomatoes).

Keeping Track

It's a smart idea to post an acceptable foods lists in your home or other places where you typically eat meals. The Atkins website (www.atkins.com) maintains multiple food lists and other tools useful to the low-carb dieter. The Atkins Carb Counter is a sixty-three-page downloadable PDF that lists the net carb content of many common foods, including generic items as well as common brand and restaurant foods. This list can be easily printed and kept in the kitchen for reference, or you can send away for a free, pocket-sized booklet to carry with you. There are also a variety of mobile phone apps that help you track the carb content of the foods you eat so you don't have to remember everything! Check out Chapter 14 for recommendations.

Foods with Labels (Packaged Foods)

If you're not in the habit of eating fresh foods and don't like to cook, and you're worried about finding foods to eat, the first thing I want you to do is go to your regular grocery store and find five *packaged* items you've never tried before that have no more than 3 g of carbs per serving. The items must have food labels (i.e., fresh meat and produce don't count).

Think it's impossible? Here's a hint: try the pickled foods section, sauces, and spreads, and the baking ingredients section. You'll be surprised by what you find!

I've said this elsewhere and it's worth repeating: approach this new eating plan with a bit of curiosity, and look to have some fun!

Calculating Net Carbs

You must learn how to calculate net carbs. We covered this in Chapter 5, but because this is probably the single most important skill needed to successfully carry out the ketogenic diet, it's worth reviewing again. You will have a very hard time finding appropriate keto foods unless you are able to calculate net carbs from a Nutrition Facts label in a snap.

The Food and Drug Administration (FDA) determines what information must be on a Nutrition Facts label and how it can be displayed. Manufacturers are required to list "total carbohydrates," as well as the sub-categories "fiber" and "sugar," but they are *not* required to list starch. You have to count grams from sugar *and* starch in your carb allotment on the ketogenic diet (remember, fiber is a freebie), but the starch grams *are missing* from the label!

This is confusing and frustrating to someone trying to avoid carbs, but there's an easy way around it. Subtract fiber from total carbs to get net carbs, and you're done. The "sugars" line is unimportant. In fact, it's best to ignore that line completely.

You are concerned only with net carbs. Net Carbs = Total Carbs – Fiber

Packaged foods are required by law to have a Nutrition Facts label and ingredient list. Use these tools to guide you when eating anything that comes in a box, can, bag, or any other container. I cannot express this enough: don't assume that particular items are carb-free, or that they are full of carbs! It's nearly impossible to tell what's in a product from looking at the front of the box. You must read the regulated labels. If you ignore them you're destined either to inadvertently eat too many carbs, or you'll just miss out on things you *can* have.

A good rule of thumb is to eats foods that contain *at most* 5 g of carbs per serving. You will find many things to eat that have much less, so read the labels!

It's helpful to know some measurement conversions when you're calculating net carbs for any foods, as some things will be given in inconvenient units.

1 cup = 16 tablespoons (dry) = 8 fluid ounces (liquid)

1 tablespoon = 3 teaspoons (dry) = ½ fluid ounce (liquid)

1 ounce = 30 grams

1 liter = 4 cups

Nuts and Seeds

Nuts and seeds are popular on the ketogenic diet because they are high in fat, moderate in protein, and low in carbs—just like the diet itself! Nuts can be eaten in many forms: raw or roasted; with or without added oil or salt; as nut/seed butters; or as ground nut/seed flours to replace wheat flour. Although the majority of the calories in nuts and seeds come from fat and protein, they are not carb-free foods. Nuts vary widely in their net carb content—cashews have three times the amount of carbs as almonds! Read the labels on nut and seed products to calculate the net carbs.

Good nut choices are:

- Almonds
- Brazil nuts
- Hazelnuts
- Macadamia nuts
- Peanuts
- Pecans
- Pine nuts
- Walnuts

Good seed choices are:

- Chia
- Flax
- Hemp
- Pumpkin
- Sesame
- Sunflower

Nut and Seed Butters

Almond butter and other similar items are a very convenient keto food, but these can be an accidental source of carbs. Many nut butters have added sugar, honey, chocolate, or other ingredients. Look only for unsweetened products. The ingredients should be the given nut (e.g., almonds) and possibly salt—and that's it. Also, some nut butters are labeled as one type (e.g., "walnut butter") but actually contain a mixture of nuts (e.g., walnuts, pecans, cashews).

Because some types of nuts have more carbs, you must read the ingredient list and calculate the net carbs.

Good options are:

- Almond butter
- Tahini (sesame seed butter)
- Coconut butter
- Peanut butter
- Sunflower seed butter (beware—many products are sweetened)
- Walnut butter (if no cashews)

Fat Types in Nuts and Seeds by Percentage

Numbers are rounded to nearest whole.

	SATURATED FAT %	MONO-UNSATURATED FAT %	POLY-UNSATURATED FAT %
Almonds	8	66	26
Brazil nuts	25	41	34
Cashews*	21	62	18
Chia seeds	11	8	81
Flaxseeds	9	19	72
Hazelnuts (filberts)	8	79	14
Macadamia nuts	16	82	2
Pecans	9	60	32
Pine nuts	9	33	59
Pistachios*	13	56	32
Pumpkin seeds	19	35	46
Sesame seeds	15	40	46
Sunflower seeds	10	40	50
Walnuts	10	14	76

Source: USDA National Nutrient Database for Standard Reference, version 26

*These are relatively high in carbs and should be consumed sparingly.

Tip

Cashews have a very high carb content, and pistachios come in second. These nuts should be avoided or consumed in very small amounts.

Non-Dairy Beverages

Non-dairy beverages are not only for drinking; they're often used in food preparation. While fluid dairy milk is a no-go on the ketogenic diet, non-dairy nut- and seed-milks are a popular keto-friendly beverage. Buy *only* unsweetened milks made from nuts (e.g., almonds) or seeds (e.g., hemp). Grain- or legume-based milks like rice or soy milk have a very high carb content. It is crucial to *read the label*, as it's often the case that (even unsweetened) products from different brands contain different ingredients, and thus different amounts of carbs. Look for the following non-dairy beverages:

- Almond milk
- Coconut milk
- Flax milk
- Hazelnut milk
- Hemp milk

Should You Count Every Carb?

Yes! But don't worry, not all of your foods need to be carbohydrate-free. Not all of your foods need to be carbohydrate-free! You'll eat many foods that have just a small amount of carbs so that when you add them up you won't eat more than 25–50 g for the day (depending on your threshold). You'll find it much easier than you think. A lot of foods have no carbs at all! Carbohydrate-free foods are much more available nowadays than ever before, thanks in part to the popularity of low-carb diets, a shifting public awareness of what constitutes a healthful diet, and the long-awaited admission of the nutrition and medical communities that carbohydrates are likely contributing significantly (and more so than fat) to the national epidemics of obesity and heart disease.

Other Beverages

Water is a mainstay of a healthful ketogenic (or any) diet. But it needn't be the only thing you drink. If you're open to trying something new, check out the carb-free beverages in your local grocery store, such as:

- Flavored water (make sure it's unsweetened)
- Seltzer (also called sparkling water, club soda, and soda water)
- Zero-calorie drinks
- Tea
- Coffee or coffee substitutes

Finding Rare Food Products

At least once a month I find a new keto-friendly product at the grocery store. Seaweed snacks, flax crackers, stevia-sweetened chocolate bars, and kale chips are popping up everywhere. The very-low-carb diet trend is gaining steam, and if you live in a large city you'll likely have an easy time finding these keto convenience foods. If you're in a smaller town you might have to hunt a little to find some of these great items, or buy them online. The resource guide at the back of the book (page 290) lists some sites where you can do so.

It's a good idea to explore the grocery and health food stores in your area. You may be surprised at what you find! And, if you don't find what you're looking for, you can ask the grocery manager if they'd be willing to carry it. This is one of the ways that new products come to the shelves—by customer request. As a time-saving measure, if you're looking for something specific and don't know if your store has it, give them a call beforehand to ask. You'll spend five minutes on the phone and may save yourself a trip!

Foods Not Suitable for the Ketogenic Diet

Thus far we've talked about the foods and food groups that, in varying amounts, make up the foundation of the ketogenic diet. The section that follows covers foods and food groups that are excluded from the diet due to their high carb content.

Fruit

Fruit is probably the thing that most people are surprised they have to give up on the ketogenic diet. "But isn't fruit healthy?" they ask. "I thought I was supposed to eat five to nine servings of fruits and vegetables per day?" Fruits contain vitamins and minerals, fiber—and a whole lot of sugar. Fruit is a tasty treat every once in a while, but sugary bananas and grapes are certainly not the same as spinach and broccoli. Fruit has very little place in the ketogenic diet at the start, although you can add low-sugar fruits in small amounts as you progress.

Some forms of fruit have a very high sugar content and should remain on your list of foods to avoid or minimize, even after you have reached your goal weight, as they pack a lot of sugar calories in each serving.

Fruit Products to Avoid

- Dried or dehydrated fruits such as raisins, dried apricots, prunes, dried pineapple slices, etc. Removing the water from fresh fruits concentrates the sugar calories so that an equal amount of dried fruit has much more sugar than the same amount of the fresh item.

- Fruit juices, including fresh-squeezed juice, which are almost entirely sugar.

- Fruits jams, jellies, and marmalades, such as strawberry jam, cranberry sauce, etc., including homemade versions.

- Freeze-dried fruits such as blueberries, raspberries, etc. These have had the water removed and only the sugar and fiber remains.

Hidden Sources of High-Carb Fruit Items

Many "trail mixes," "energy mixes," or "nut mixes" contain an assortment of nuts and dried fruit. Small squares of unidentifiable sweetness are likely cubed and dried pineapple or dates. Look closely at the contents of the bag when purchasing these items to avoid those with added fruit. And if you end up with a fruit-containing product, don't cheat! You can just eat around them.

Fresh vegetable juices are generally not suitable for the beginning ketogenic dieter. Keep in mind that many juices that are labeled "Green" or "Vegetable" also contain fruit (e.g., apple, grape) to enhance the sweetness. These may be very high in carbs.

Grains

Grains aren't suitable for the ketogenic diet. Even a small amount of grains will put you over your carb allotment rather quickly. **Avoid them completely**.

Any food made from wheat, rice, oats, cornmeal, barley, or another cereal grain is a considered a grain product. Bread, pasta, oatmeal, breakfast cereals, tortillas, grits, and other grain products have a very high carbohydrate content.

Keeping in mind that grains are not permitted, here are examples of common grains and grain products:

Amaranth	Grits
Barley	Macaroni
Bread	Millet
Brown rice	Muesli
Buckwheat	Noodles
Bulgur (cracked wheat)	Oatmeal
Cereal	Pasta
Cornmeal	Pita
Corn tortillas	Popcorn
Couscous	Pretzels
Crackers	Quinoa
Flour	Rice
	Rolled oats

Rye	Tortillas
Sorghum	Triticale
Spaghetti	Wheat flakes

Source: USDA, "What Foods Are in the Grains Group?" http://www.choosemyplate.gov/food-groups/grains.html. Last accessed September 1, 2014.

Tip: Avoid ALL Pasta Varieties

There are dozens of varieties of pasta made from different types of flour, and it can be tempting to think that these alternatives are low-carb. Not so. Traditional pasta is made with a type of wheat flour called *semolina*, and you may see that word written on the label. Other typical varieties include whole wheat, spinach, tri-color, and egg pasta; and newer products like corn, rice, or black bean pasta are aimed at consumers with allergies to wheat. Regardless of the type of grain, the bulk of the calories in these products come from starch, and none are suitable for the ketogenic diet. If you want to cook a keto friendly noodle dish, look for carb-free kelp or tofu noodles in the dairy case.

Gluten Lurks in Places Other Than Bread

Although most people consider "gluten" to be synonymous with "bread," it is important to know that wheat flour is not the only place where gluten is found. If you're under the impression that the ketogenic diet will help you avoid gluten, you're only partially correct. Gluten is not forbidden on the ketogenic diet. Although eliminating bread and most processed or packaged foods (as recommended on the ketogenic diet) will knock a large portion of the gluten out of your diet, there will still very likely be gluten containing items in your pantry. Soy sauce is a common culprit, as are other Asian sauces, as well as marinades, soups, processed meats, and many jarred foods that may pass criteria for the ketogenic diet. Gluten doesn't necessarily come in the form of carbohydrate foods, either (in fact, gluten itself is a protein). If you want to learn about hidden sources of gluten in foods and how to avoid them, visit the Celiac Disease Foundation website at www.celiac.org for a wealth of resources on the subject.

Starchy Vegetables

These contain a lot of carbohydrate in the form of—you guessed it—starch. They also contain sugar, a small amount of protein, and almost no fat. *Starchy vegetables are not allowed on the ketogenic diet.*

Net Carb Content in Common Preparations of Selected Starchy Vegetables

ITEM	AMOUNT	NET CARBS
Rutabagas	1 cup	8.5 g
Carrots, raw*	1 cup	8.7 g
Pumpkin	1 cup	9.3 g
Beets	1 cup	13.5 g
Peas	1 cup	14 g
Butternut squash	1 cup, cubed	15 g
Acorn squash	1 cup, cubed	20 g
Corn on the cob	1 ear	22 g
Boiled white potato	1 medium potato	25 g
Corn kernels	1 cup	30 g
Baked sweet potato	1 large potato	31 g

Mashed potatoes	1 cup	34 g
Plantains	1 cup, sliced	44 g
Mashed sweet potato	1 cup	50 g

Source. USDA National Nutrient Database for Standard Reference, version 26

*Carb content given for foods in their cooked form, except for carrots.

Beans and Legumes

As with fruit, this food group can cause some confusion to the ketogenic dieter. It's true that beans and legumes are a good source of protein, fiber, and some vitamins and minerals. But they are also very high in carbohydrate and should be avoided, at least to start. Examples are:

- Black beans
- Navy beans
- Kidney beans
- Garbanzo beans
- Lentils
- Split peas
- Chickpeas
- Lima beans
- Fava beans
- Pinto beans

Tip

Look out for foods made out of beans, such as hummus (a dip made of chickpeas), vegetarian burgers, and unidentifiable dips.

Fructose and Fat Storage

Fructose is a type of sugar that's gotten a lot of negative attention in recent years for being part of the infamous, ubiquitous industrial sweetener, high-fructose corn syrup (HFCS). But did you know that fructose is also a substantial part of good old table sugar (aka sucrose)? High-fructose corn syrup comes in two common forms: a mixture that is 55 percent fructose (the rest is glucose and water), and one that is 42 percent fructose. By comparison, table sugar is 50 percent fructose and 50 percent glucose.

Fructose is similar to glucose in shape and size, but it appears to be used differently by the body. Like glucose, fructose is sent to the liver for metabolic processing after it passes through the gut. But while glucose heads off on a journey through the bloodstream, ultimately to be used up for energy by cells all over the body (that is, in a person who's not on the ketogenic diet), fructose stays put in the liver, where it is converted easily to fat. This is one reason why scientists are beginning to suspect that excess fructose consumption may lead to rapid weight gain. Moreover, while the body does require glucose, as we have seen, for the brain and nervous system, there is no biological need for fructose—and prior to the industrial production of sugar, human exposure to fructose was very limited. Now, fructose has become widely available in sweeteners and all kinds of processed foods, so people are eating a lot more of it, and thus consuming a lot more sugar calories in general.

Although many experts debate the impact of fructose on the body's metabolism, everyone agrees that overconsumption of sugar calories is exceedingly unhealthy.

Sugar and Sweeteners

It should be rather obvious by now that sugar in any form is forbidden on the ketogenic diet. There are dozens if not hundreds of types of caloric (carb-containing) sweeteners made out of sugar or other substances, and it's nearly impossible to name them or remember them all. Your best bet is to learn the common ones, and of course, check the label of any product for net carbs.

Common household sweeteners:

- Sugar
- Honey (including raw honey)
- Molasses
- Maple syrup
- Agave syrup
- Corn syrup
- Rice syrup

Some sweeteners used in processed foods have unfamiliar names. Use the general rules below to help you figure out if an item contains sugar.

- Anything with the word "syrup," including high-fructose corn syrup, glucose-fructose syrup, pomegranate syrup, etc.
- Any word ending in "ose," including sucrose, dextrose, saccharose, etc.
- Anything with the word "sugar," including raw sugar, coconut sugar, invert sugar, etc.
- Anything with the word "cane," including cane crystals, dehydrated cane juice, evaporated cane juice, etc.

- Fruit juice concentrate
- Maltodextrin

Is there such a thing as "healthy" sugar? Not really. Sugar can be extracted from sugar cane, beets, corn, coconut, and many other crops. Although some sugars are marketed as being "healthier," they all turn into glucose in your blood. Sugar should not be eaten, regardless of the source.

Achieving sweetness without sugar

You may think that by removing sugar from your diet you'll be eliminating all sweetness, too. But that's not so! Consider that processed foods depend on industrial ingredients such as "invert sugar" for their sweetness, but home cooks certainly don't use invert sugar! In the same way, there is a different set of sweet ingredients available to you. You'll have the option to use alternative sweeteners such as erythritol and stevia (see section on alternative sweeteners on page 187) if you'd like to add a sweet note to foods. After you've lost some weight you'll decide whether you want to increase your carb allotment, and you may include fruit, or even find some room for a drop of honey or maple syrup in certain recipes.

CHAPTER 8

Meal Options

Preparing Your Pantry

Successful keto cooking is easy once you have the right ingredients. If you're an avid cook you probably already have many of these items in your kitchen.

Oils

Get a variety of oils for different uses. Some types to keep on hand:

- **Olive oil**. Ideal for salad dressings and light sautéing at low temperatures. Don't allow olive oil to smoke, as it damages the fat.

- **Coconut oil**. Stable at high temperatures and great for roasting vegetables in the oven; sautéing meat, chicken or tofu; or scrambling eggs. It's also fantastic in keto desserts to add creaminess and sweetness.

- **Avocado oil**. Like olive oil, this oil is high in mono-unsaturated fat. Use it for cold preparations or for cooking, especially at times of year when you can't find ripe avocados.

- **Flaxseed oil**. Another high omega-3 oil that should be stored in the refrigerator. Use in smoothies rather than for food preparation.

- **Sesame oil**. A highly flavorful oil, especially the toasted variety. It comes in small bottles and you won't use a lot—just add a touch to dishes near the end of cooking for a nutty, earthy flavor.

Flavored oils using herbs or spices are a nice addition to meals, but they can also be quite expensive and may not be very fresh if purchased. Fortunately, you can easily make these on your own using plain olive oil as your base. Common types are: garlic, rosemary, and red chile pepper. If using fresh herbs or garlic you must blanche them for one minute in boiling water before using (dry herbs can be used directly). Then, heat the blanched ingredients in olive oil on low flame for two to three minutes or until fragrant. Use right away, or let cool and pour into a glass bottle for later use. Store in a cool, dark cabinet or in the refrigerator.

Salt and Pepper

Salt and pepper are important flavoring agents that can greatly improve the taste of your food.

Salt. Salt is essential for delicious eating. Salt doesn't just add a "salty" taste; it actually enhances the flavors in a food. You'll also need more salt on the ketogenic diet, so keep some on the table to add to meals while you're eating. If all you've ever known is table salt (the type that costs about $0.89 in the grocery store and tends to have an unpleasant metallic flavor), then you may not think that salt is so great. Use *sea salt* instead, which is fresh and vibrant-tasting, and rich with minerals. Basic sea salt costs about $3–$4 for a large container that lasts for months. Salting meats and chicken before cooking, adding salt to your vegetables in their pan, and sprinkling salt on salads will greatly improve the flavor of your meals.

Pepper. As with salt, if you've only ever tried the ground stuff sitting for years in a pepper shaker that makes you sneeze when you use it, then you may not be so excited about pepper. Use *fresh cracked pepper* instead, which has a bright peppery taste and gives a new layer of flavor to a lot of foods. Pepper meats before cooking for some spice and texture (freshly ground pepper grains are bigger). Fresh pepper is a nice addition to salads and simple vegetables such as roasted asparagus.

Dry Spices and Herbs

There are hundreds of dry spices that any interested cook can use to flavor a dish. If you're open to exploring new spices, check out a local spice shop or specialty foods store. Indian or Southeast Asian markets are also great places for finding new spices.

At minimum, keep a basic array of spices on hand, including:

- **Basil, rosemary, thyme, parsley, and oregano.** These are just some of the dry green herbs that are great for meat or poultry marinades, for use in sauces, for sprinkling over vegetables before baking, and a host of other uses.

- **Herbs de Provence.** This is a mixture of green herbs that sometimes includes lavender; it's very aromatic and makes a nice addition to omelets.

- **Paprika.** This bright red spice is underutilized. Paprika can be used to add flavor to just about anything. Sweet paprika is not exactly "sweet" tasting but rather a mixture of sweet, sour, and earthy; use it with chicken, eggs, and tofu. Smoked paprika is quite smoky and pairs nicely with meat.

- **Cayenne.** Cayenne or ground red pepper is *hot*. Use just a pinch to spice up salsas, omelets, tomato sauce, or meat marinades.

- **Cumin.** Cumin comes in either seed or powder form and is a common ingredient in many non-American cuisines. It's often blended into dips (like baba ghanoush) and sauces (like salsas).

- **Chili powder.** Unlike cayenne, most chili powders are mild in flavor (although some can be hot). Chili imparts an earthy flavor to foods.

- **Red pepper flakes.** These are also *hot*; use carefully. Red pepper flakes go great with hearty green vegetables (kale, broccoli, rapini) sautéed in olive oil and garlic.

- **Cinnamon.** Because it's often paired with sweet things, many people think cinnamon itself is sweet. It's not; it's actually rather bitter. It gives a pungent, spicy kick to smoothies and keto desserts, but don't overdo it thinking you'll bring out some sweetness—the more you add, the harsher the flavor.

- **Ginger.** Powdered ginger is a handy substitute for fresh ginger. It's nice with turmeric in meat marinades, or for spiciness in smoothies.

- **Turmeric.** A brilliant yellow spice used in Indian curries. It has a bright, slightly gingery flavor. Turmeric has tremendous medicinal properties; it's used as an antiviral, anti-inflammatory, and anti-cancer agent in Chinese and Indian (Ayurvedic) medicine traditions. Many people don't know how to use turmeric, but it's quite simple: add it to scrambled eggs, sprinkle it on salads, and include it in meat marinades.

Although dry spices and herbs are not carb-free, these ingredients are used in such small amounts that they shouldn't cause much concern during your ketogenic diet.

Net Carb Contents in One Teaspoon of Selected Dry Spices and Herbs

SPICE	NET CARBS
Thyme	0.2 g
Sage	0.2 g
Marjoram	0.2 g
Oregano	0.3 g
Rosemary	0.3 g
Parsley	0.3 g
Chili powder	0.4 g
Paprika	0.4 g
Cayenne	0.5 g
Nutmeg	0.6 g
Cinnamon	0.7 g
Cloves	0.7 g
Black pepper	0.9 g
Ginger powder	1 g
Turmeric powder	1.3 g
Onion powder	1.5 g
Garlic powder	2 g

Source: USDA National Nutrient Database for Standard Reference, version 26

Fresh Herbs

In addition to dry herbs mentioned above, a variety of fresh herbs can add vibrant flavors to a host of dishes. Unlike dry spices, you must buy these fresh, refrigerate, and use them quickly. They range in net carb content from less than ½ g to about 1 g per cup.

Big leafy herbs like basil, cilantro, dill, mint, and parsley should be purchased fresh and green, with no brown spots. Store refrigerated and use within a week. These can be used in large amounts (e.g., ¼ to ½ cup, chopped) for a nice aromatic flavor in salads or vegetable dishes (try a mixture of chopped basil and mint in a salad—yum!). Mint is great for flavoring water or unsweetened tea.

Smaller fresh herbs like rosemary, thyme, and oregano are sold in packages and can last about 3 weeks in the refrigerator. They have a stronger flavor and should be used in smaller amounts; about 1 tablespoon of chopped rosemary goes well in meat marinades or to flavor cauliflower mash.

Condiments and Sauces

You should be delighted to learn that many sauces and condiments are low-carb or carb-free. However, many others are carb-heavy! The key to success here is to *read labels and choose carefully*.

Condiments and sauces are important flavoring agents for any diet. You'll need the following:

Tomato sauce. Tomato sauce *can* be suitable for the ketogenic diet, but be aware that many jarred tomato sauces have *a lot* of added sugar. Some, though, have very little or none at all, and the taste doesn't suffer. It's worth reading the labels on those at your grocery store to find the lowest carb option rather than buying one with added sugar and wasting your 25–50 g carb allotment that way.

Vinegars. Vinegars are essential to mix with oil for dressings and marinades. But keep in mind that some vinegars can be high in carbs. Mix sweeter varieties, like balsamic, with less sweet types, like white wine, to get a mix that's not too sour and also won't blow your carb allotment.

How to Make a Marinade in Under Two Minutes

The flavor of cooked proteins (meats, poultry, shrimp, tofu) is greatly improved by marinating them for as little as thirty minutes. You'll notice huge payoff on the tastiness scale for just one minute's worth of prep work. The same trick works for vegetables if you're baking them (sautéed vegetables are usually flavored during cooking).

1. Get out a deep dish or bowl big enough to hold whatever you're marinating.

2. Put some oil in it (any type).

3. Put the same amount of vinegar, lemon, or lime juice in it.

4. Add any herb you like (rosemary, thyme, etc.).

5. Put the food in the dish and massage for a few seconds with the marinade, then let sit for thirty minutes or up to several hours in the refrigerator before cooking.

How to Make Vinaigrette in Under Two Minutes

Bottled salad dressing is expensive and usually contains sugar and/or starch. It takes less than two minutes to make your own, and you can keep it for a couple of weeks in a jar in the refrigerator.

1. Pour ½ cup of vinegar in a blender (mix vinegar types if you'd like).

2. Add 1 tablespoon of Dijon mustard (this should not contain a sweetener; check the label).

3. Add 1 teaspoon of sea salt and, if using, herbs, shallots, or spices.

4. Blend.

5. Add 1 cup of olive or other cold prep oil.

6. Blend again.

7. Bottle and refrigerate.

Asian sauces. Asian sauces can give the all-important "umami," or meaty, flavor to foods. Adding soy sauce to a marinade or sprinkling it on proteins or vegetables while cooking will bring bland dishes to the next level. (Don't add too much or the food will turn out salty.) Some Asian sauces have a citrusy or sour flavor that adds even more complexity to your dish. Keep these in your kitchen! But be choosy: Asian sauces run the gamut from less than 1 g of carbs per serving to 20 g! Carb-heavy products have sugar, sweeteners, and starches, and ambiguous names like "stir-fry sauce," make it impossible to know the ingredients. Don't write off the whole category or you will be missing out on a range of fantastic flavors. Just read labels and choose carefully.

Salsas. These are most often a mix of tomatoes and other vegetables (e.g., onions, peppers), vinegar, and spices, with or without sugar. Tomato salsa and green salsa or salsa verde (made with tomatillos) can be used in limited amounts depending on their ingredients. Salsas are wonderful on egg or fish dishes. You can also make your own!

Mustard. Plain Dijon is useful for sauces and salad dressing. Herbed Dijon mustards are delicious on burgers instead of ketchup, which is usually sweetened. Avoid mustards with honey or sugar, such as "Honey Dijon."

Mayonnaise. Made of eggs and oil, mayonnaise is perfect for the ketogenic diet! But watch out, because some products may have sweeteners. Vegan mayonnaise is made of a mixture of oils and is usually also carb-free.

Pickled things. Many pickled items are low enough in carbs and used in small enough amounts that they fit into a keto diet plan. As always, check the labels.

Flour Substitutes for Baking

There is a great variety of nut and seed flours in the baking section of the grocery store that can substitute for wheat flour. If you've never had reason to look for these then you probably don't know they exist. Take fifteen minutes the next time you're shopping to familiarize yourself with these flours—and *make sure to read the labels!* Flours made from grains other than wheat, such as rice or millet, and those made from starches, such as potato and arrowroot, are extremely high in carbs and are *not* appropriate for keto dieting.

The following are some good pantry basics:

- Almond flour is a great substitute for wheat flour. It can be used in most baking recipes, for "breading" meat or fish, as a binder in meatballs, or to thicken a sauce or smoothie. The flavor is a touch sweeter than that of wheat flour.

- Flax meal is coarser than a powder and is a good substitute for bread crumbs. Use as a "breading" or crust for chicken, fish, or cauliflower, and add to smoothies for extra texture and a dose of omega-3 fats.

- Coconut flour is very fine and may have a mildly sweet or just coconutty taste, depending on your palate. It's a good ingredient for baking, although much less coconut flour is needed than wheat flour in a given recipe, and extra eggs are usually also needed for volume and texture. It takes some practice and experimentation to learn the best proportion for your recipes.

There are a variety of other flours made from nuts (e.g., hazelnut) and seeds (e.g., sesame seed) that can be useful substitutes for you. Be aware that recipes made with these flours in lieu of wheat flour will not produce identical results. You will be most successful if you're willing to experiment a bit with the different flours to learn how they add texture, volume, and flavor to foods. Do some research on cooking blogs (keto, paleo, and gluten-free baking sites are a smart choice) and in cookbooks devoted to the subject.

Tip

Unlike wheat flour, nut and seed flours should be stored in the refrigerator because the fats in them can spoil easily.

Alternative Sweeteners

Alternative sweeteners come in natural and artificial (synthetically produced) types, and they are a mixed bag. With regard to taste, the two types have similar, shall we say, "challenges." While they add some sweetness with very few or no carbs, many have an "off" taste that is displeasing to those who notice it. Fortunately, not everyone notices, and many who do eventually stop noticing—especially once their inner sugar fiend is laid to rest. A lot of baked goods made with alternative sweeteners taste the same as or quite similar to those made with sugar, and you can usually make the switch in sauces, dressings, smoothies, and other items that call for a dash of sweetness without any noticeable difference.

With regard to health, there are some big differences between natural and artificial sweeteners. The potential negative health effects of artificial sweeteners has been an area of some controversy for decades. You are probably familiar with many of these, such as aspartame (sold as NutraSweet or Equal) and saccharin (commonly used in soft drinks). At worst, some of these chemicals cause cancer in laboratory animals. At best, they're more or less safe for humans in small amounts. Evidence continues to surface on both sides, so it's hard to say how safe these ingredients really are.

This is a shaky foundation from which to make dietary recommendations. The major problem is this: being overweight also increases one's risk of cancer. In a perfect world, we wouldn't love sweetness so much and this question would be moot. But in the real world we sometimes want sweet things, and artificial sweeteners, risky as they may be, are a calorie-free way to get your fix.

Natural sweeteners are a different ballgame entirely. The general consensus is that these products do not pose a threat to human health. The two main types are sugar alcohols and stevia.

Sugar alcohols as a group are less sweet than sugar. Sugar alcohols are not completely digested, so they contribute fewer carbs than sugar—but they are not carb-free! The digested portion converts to sugar, so you must count these in your carb intake. Sugar alcohols are suitable in small amounts on the ketogenic diet. Xylitol and erythritol are commonly use in keto baked goods and keto desserts. Unfortunately, the incomplete digestion of these ingredients can cause gas, bloating, and diarrhea if they are consumed in large amounts, which is a convenient disincentive to overeating them!

Stevia is made from a leaf and contains no carbs or calories at all. Some people are put off by the taste of stevia (particularly the aftertaste), and others don't mind it. There is considerable research underway to find a better-tasting stevia extract, and you can be assured that in the next few years you'll find more (and hopefully improved) stevia products on the market.

Stevia chocolate bars can take care of a chocolate craving with very little damage in the carb department, although you might have to suffer through the aftertaste.

Novel Packaged Foods Suitable for the Ketogenic Diet

One of the biggest challenges on the ketogenic diet is that typical "convenience" or packaged foods are pretty much off limits. This is sort of a good thing, since it reduces snacking and forces you to have healthier meals, which ultimately aids weight loss. Sometimes, though, you need a little convenience. Thanks in part to the paleo diet and the growing awareness of gluten-intolerance, a host of very-low-carb foods are coming out on the market that will make your life on keto much easier.

Chia seeds. Chia seeds are tiny (commonly black in color) seeds that swell when placed in water, which makes them useful as thickeners. I use chia seeds in my smoothies to thicken them, and for chia pudding as a dessert (see recipes). Chia seeds also add a nice textural element if you sprinkle them dry over foods.

Flax crackers. These are sort of a keto lifesaver. They stand in perfectly for wheat crackers. They're crunchy and delicious, and since they're made of flax they have only 1 g of carbs per serving. These should be available at your local upscale grocery or health food store. The brand Dr. In the Kitchen makes them in five flavors and in the familiar size and shapes of crackers. Foods Alive makes a variety of flavors, including a ginger snap which is just sweet enough that you can satisfy a sweet craving without going over your carb limit, and an Italian zest flavor that tastes very much like pizza.

Tip

Two Moms in the Raw Pesto Sea Crackers are a terrific substitute for croutons. These are lighter and thinner than flax crackers, and less suitable for holding heavy toppings like cheese or nut butters. They are best crumbled and added to salads for a nice crunch!

Kelp noodles. These are made of seaweed and salt, and they contain no carbs, fat, or protein. Kelp noodles are 100 percent calorie free. They are also flavorless, so they're more or less just a vehicle for sauce. You can use them like spaghetti. Tofu noodles are similar to kelp noodles but sometimes contain a couple of carb grams per serving.

Coconut (and coconut oil, coconut butter, coconut cream, etc.). If foods could be royalty, coconut would be crowned queen of the ketogenic diet. First, many people find that coconut is delicious. Second, coconut is mostly fat, and a high proportion of that fat is in the form of medium chain triglycerides (MCTs), which enhance ketosis. Third, there is a huge variety of products made from coconut that are useful on the ketogenic diet: coconut oil for cooking and especially for baking; coconut butter and cream for making keto desserts; coconut flour to use as a substitute for wheat flour; and plain (unsweetened) shredded coconut meat for toppings or to use in smoothies. The only part of the coconut you don't want is the water: it's too high in carbs.

Cacao powder. If you've always been a chocolate lover it's a good idea to buy some cacao powder, unsweetened, of course. You can add it to smoothies and keto desserts if you need to get your chocolate fix. You can also add it to spice mixtures when cooking meats.

Seaweed snacks. These are available in any Asian grocery and some supermarkets. They're strips of seasoned seaweed. You get the crunchy, salty fix without all the carbs that would come in many other snack foods. They usually come in single serving packs that are 1 g of carbs each.

Fermented vegetables. These are in the cheese case in the grocery store. In fermentation, bacteria are added to a food that has some sugar, and the bacteria eat the sugar, turning it into acid and giving the food a sour flavor. Because of this, fermented vegetables have less sugar than fresh vegetables and you can eat small amounts of some varieties that you'd avoid fresh, such as carrots and beets. There are many kinds of fermented vegetables, with Korean cabbage (kimchi) and German cabbage (sauerkraut) being the widely known varieties. Fermented vegetables have unique flavors, and they can add some brightness and lightness to fat-heavy keto meals. Note: Do not mistake regular "pickled vegetables" for fermented vegetables, as regular pickles more often have sugar added.

Kale chips. These are the twenty-first century potato chip. They come in a variety of flavors and can be addictive. Be careful! You can only eat a small amount if you want to stay under your carb allotment.

Planning a Keto Meal

Develop Some Carb-Counting Expertise

You've heard me say many times that you must learn how to
estimate the amount of carbs in the foods you're eating and
calculate the net carbs from nutritional labels when available. You simply can't skip developing this skill and expect
to do well on the ketogenic diet! I strongly encourage you
to learn more about the nutrient content of the foods you
eat as you move through changing your diet. Use the list
in "Food for Thought" on page 196, as well as the "Components of a Keto Meal" on page 194 as a starting place.
Carefully read the chapter "What Can I Eat" on page 141
to learn some of the basics, download a nutrition-tracking
app or print out a food nutrient reference list to keep with
you at all times, and visit the sites in the resource section of
this book to keep up with new low-carb food products and
get tips from like-minded ketogenic dieters. *Do not dismiss
these steps as unnecessary.* Your journey with the ketogenic
diet may begin with this book, but if you want to maintain
a low-carb lifestyle and the weight loss that accompanies
it, you will want to develop a better understanding of food.

Whether you become a "food expert" is up to you, but at the very least you'll want to know more about nutrition than the average person!

How Fat Looks on the Plate

Although most of the calories in your meals will come from fat, most of the visible "stuff" on your plate will not be fat. Remember, fat has more than twice the calories as the same amount of carbs or protein, so you will not need to eat as much of it (in terms of volume) to feel satisfied.

If this isn't crystal clear, consider the following example:

Imagine 1 cup of cooked spinach.
(This is a carbohydrate.)
Imagine 1 cup of diced chicken.
(This is a protein.)
Imagine 1 cup of olive oil.
(This is a fat.)

Do you think you can swallow the full amount of each of these? If not, which one do you think you would have a hard time getting down? Right, it's the olive oil.

You'll also notice that fat doesn't take up as much visual space as carbs or protein. Consider the foods mentioned above; even if you did pour one cup of olive oil over a plate of spinach and chicken, the oil would pool underneath those foods and wouldn't make much of an appearance, so to speak. You don't usually "see" the oil in which you've cooked your food, or the dressing clinging to the leaves of lettuce in your salad. For this reason, it's practical to build meals around a protein item and a non-starchy vegetable—the things we see—and then add on fats as side items (e.g., avocado), cooking oils (e.g., coconut oil), toppings (e.g., sesame seeds), sauces (e.g., lemon-butter sauce), and dressings (e.g., creamy Italian).

Components of a Keto Meal

1. Protein

You will probably have a main protein item for two of three meals a day (if you have three meals). You may easily skip protein for snacks and smaller meals.

For full meals, have a nice piece of fish, chicken, tofu, pork, beef, or other meat. It doesn't have to be just a plain slab of meat. You can have grilled shrimp on skewers, bison meatballs, or diced fish in tartare. Four to six ounces is a good amount to start with, and you can have more if you are a large man, in intensive physical training, or if you simply find this amount isn't enough—but pay attention to your symptoms and make sure you're not preventing ketosis by overloading on protein. Eggs are another major source of protein, as is protein powder you may use in smoothies.

If you're just having a snack rather than a meal, or a meal based on low-carb vegetables, then the protein may not be the center of your plate. For example, cheese and cucumbers, almond butter and celery sticks, or kelp noodles with pesto all have small amounts of protein, although the protein component is less obvious.

2. Non-Starchy Vegetables

Remember, you'll use your daily carb allotment of 25–50 g almost entirely on non-starchy vegetables. These foods are your main source of fiber, water-soluble vitamins, and many minerals, and it's wise to include them right up to your daily limit. Plan to add a side of roasted or sautéed vegetables or a small salad to your proteins. Sautéed broccoli or cauli-flower, roasted asparagus, or mixed greens are a great start. If you have time to make a main salad, use a base of low-carb greens like spinach or arugula, and add protein and fats to round out the meal. If you have less time, add some cucumber or zucchini sticks to your plate, or throw some handfuls of spinach leaves into the pan as you cook some eggs or meat. Check the vegetable chart on page 145 for carb counts.

3. Fats

Make sure to have two or more sources of fats in all of your meals, and at least one in all of your snacks. Food items that are mainly fat include avocado, nuts or nut butters, seeds, cheese or cream, bacon, and egg yolk. You can also count the fat that comes in fatty cuts of meat or fatty fish. It's easy to include these foods in your meals: use sliced avocado to accompany meat, sprinkle seeds on top of your food (both chicken and broccoli are delicious covered with ses-ame seeds), melt cheese onto roasted vegetables, etc. The harder part is remembering to add oils and fat-rich sauces to your meals. Use a variety of oils or butter for cooking protein items or vegetables. Pour pan drippings directly over cooked foods, or add butter or heavy cream to make a sauce for the same purpose. Add butter to vegetables once they're on your plate, if you'd like. Make or buy mayonnaise, cream or cheese dips, guacamole, and oil-based spreads to add to your plate for dipping any item whatsoever. Use full fat salad dressings for salads. If you find you've somehow prepared a meal that's lacking in fat, just drizzle some olive oil over your finished dish.

Remember don't forget the fat!

While you don't necessarily need to include protein or non-starchy vegetables at every meal, it rarely—if ever—makes sense to have a ketogenic meal without fat. I can only think of a few cases in which you might do so: munching on celery sticks or cucumber slices alone, or eating a skinless chicken breast with nothing on it. While you can get away with this every once in a while, it's not ideal for maintaining ketosis and you will likely become hungry again in a short while. It's a much better idea to add some fat-containing dipping sauces, dressings, mayonnaise, and so forth to these snacks.

Food for Thought

Foods to Eat and Drink

You should be eating fats, protein foods, and non-starchy vegetables such as:

- Oils
- Avocado
- Butter/cream/cheese
- Meats
- Poultry
- Fish/Seafood
- Tofu
- Eggs

- Nuts/Seeds
- Kale, spinach, and other leafy greens
- Broccoli, cauliflower, and cabbage
- Salad vegetables
- Mushrooms

You may also consume "non-nutritive" foods and beverages provided they contain no caloric sweeteners (calorie-free alternative sweeteners are acceptable) like coffee, tea, and seltzer water.

Foods NOT to Eat

Do not eat any sweet or starchy foods. Avoid sugar in any form, all grains, all starchy vegetables, and most dairy products (cheese and heavy cream are acceptable). Here is a sampling of foods to avoid:

- sugar
- honey
- syrup
- juice
- bread
- flour

- rice
- oats
- potatoes
- corn
- fruit

Breakfast

Many people find it hard to eat a healthy breakfast *regardless* of the type of diet they follow. Maybe it's because we tend to rush in the mornings and resort to grabbing something (typically unhealthy) on the way to work. Also, breakfast is often associated with carbohydrate-heavy foods like cereal, bagels, and muffins that are certainly not acceptable fare on the ketogenic diet. The long-standing fear of fat and cholesterol is probably another factor, since savory breakfast foods like eggs and bacon tend to contain both. So now that you're on a fat-happy diet you're wondering if it's eggs and bacon every morning, right? Well, you can certainly eat those, but I urge you to aim for a bit more variety than that!

Here are my top five favorite keto breakfasts:

1. **Eggs**. Yes, eggs, but don't be boring about it!
   And meat needn't always accompany these oval
   delights. Sauté some onions and mushrooms, or
   whatever non-starchy vegetables you have on
   hand (asparagus, chopped broccoli, spinach, etc.),
   in some olive or coconut oil. Then, while you're
   whisking your eggs, sprinkle in a nice array of
   spices. Turmeric adds an earthy punch; oregano or
   thyme lend some herbal freshness; and chile flakes,
   black pepper, or cayenne bring some heat. Use a
   liberal amount of salt. Think of the eggs as your
   canvas, and use spices and herbs to take the flavor
   up a notch. You can whisk in some heavy cream
   if you want them fluffier. It's easiest to pour the
   eggs into the vegetables as they sauté, and just
   scramble it all up. Or, you can fold the ingredients
   into a nice omelet. Top with salsa, sour cream, or
   avocado if you're in the mood. If you're still hungry,
   have a handful of walnuts, and next time, use more
   oil. Another egg favorite is fried eggs, avocado,
   bacon, and aioli, with a side of salad greens.

2. **Leftovers from dinner the night before**. A nice
   thing about the ketogenic diet is that you stop
   craving a "sweet" meal in the morning. Once that
   happens, breakfast stops being a special meal
   category and you can pretty much eat whatever
   you want in the a.m. Sometimes, dinner is so
   delicious that if you have leftovers you will spend
   the next day waiting for dinner just so you can have
   a second helping. But on keto you don't feel weird
   about just waking up and eating it. I can say from

personal experience that rosemary lemon chicken with aioli and asparagus is a very nice breakfast!

3. **Little open-faced sandwiches of cheddar or Swiss cheese on slices of baby cucumber or flax crackers.** Sprinkle the cucumbers with salt before topping with cheese. I often eat these for breakfast or snack and they are extraordinarily satisfying. It may sound like a light breakfast, but do you remember eating crackers and cheese for breakfast on occasion and thinking that was enough? Or a bagel with cream cheese? We're just swapping out the bread for cucumber or flax crackers.

4. **A smoothie.** This is not the quickest breakfast, in my opinion, because you have to blend everything and then clean the blender. Personally, I find it's easier to scramble up some eggs, but many people consider smoothies a very convenient breakfast. Either way, do some experimenting with keto-friendly smoothies. Try different combinations of unsweetened almond milk or hemp milk, low-carb protein powder, some spinach leaves for volume, hemp seeds, chia seeds, flax powder, coconut butter, almond butter, avocado, stevia, cinnamon, ginger, etc. There are endless combinations. When you find one you love, post it on a keto discussion board for the rest of us to enjoy!

5. **Plain Icelandic or Greek yogurt with a giant spoonful of almond butter.** The contrast of the cool, creamy yogurt with the hot-and-heavy almond butter is delicious. Make sure that your choice of yogurt is very low in carbs—5 g per 6 oz

is about as high as you want to go. If you find the taste of plain yogurt to be too sour, mix half a container of plain with half a container of a *lightly* flavored or sweetened variety, like vanilla or coconut. Alternatively, you can choose a smooth tub cheese in place of the yogurt, which will be richer but less sour. Fromage blanc, cottage cheese, and quark are good choices. If you're looking for some crunch you can top with chopped nuts and seeds, or have a side of flax crackers, and that should do the trick.

Breakfast Shopping List

If you typically eat lunch and dinner out and breakfast is the only meal you need to shop for, make sure these are at the top of your grocery list:

- Eggs
- An assortment of non-starchy vegetables such as asparagus, tomato, spinach, onions, peppers, mushrooms, etc.
- Baby salad greens or spinach
- Sliced meats, bacon, or sausages (without sweeteners)
- Avocado
- Smoked fish, such as lox or whitefish
- Strained yogurt
- Hard and soft cheeses
- Seeds, such as chia and flax
- Almond or other nut or seed milk (unsweetened)

- Low-carb protein powder
- Condiments, such as hot sauce, sour cream, and salsas (without sugar)
- Smoothie ingredients, such as cacao powder and cinnamon
- Spices, such as smoked paprika, turmeric, and Herbs de Provence

Snacks

In reality, on the ketogenic diet you may not feel like eating three times a day. You may have breakfast in the early part of the day and one other meal later on. If you're eating in a hurry during the workday, you'll probably opt for something closer to an afternoon snack rather than a meal. Here are some of my favorite keto snacks:

- Flax crackers and sliced cheese
- Celery sticks and almond butter
- Avocado and tomato slices with salt
- Mixed nuts and seeds in unsweetened almond milk (perhaps with cinnamon, stevia, half a cup of berries, etc.)
- Cucumber sticks and tahini
- Broccoli/broccolini with baba ghanoush
- Asparagus with aioli dipping sauce
- Endive with herbed goat cheese
- Sliced Persian cucumber and Swiss cheese "sandwiches"
- Flax crackers and goat Gouda, with or without red bell pepper spread

- Mixed vegetables with guacamole
- Prosciutto and cheese roll-ups
- Zucchini sticks with red pepper spread
- Boiled eggs with salt
- Celery sticks and cream cheese
- Fromage blanc or Greek yogurt with chopped walnuts
- Seaweed snacks, any flavor
- Mixed nuts (excluding cashews and pistachios)

Lunch and Dinner

There isn't necessarily a big difference between lunch and dinner meals on the ketogenic diet. Unless you're just eating a snack, you'll organize your plate as described earlier in "Components of a Keto Meal" on page 194. Make a protein item and vegetables, and add a good amount of fat. It's convenient to bake enough chicken or tofu for two or three meals all at once, so that you have leftovers during the week. When you're feeling indulgent, broil a steak, or cook up some beef or bison meatballs. Aim to eat fish twice a week.

Here's six of my favorite ketogenic lunches and dinners:

1. **Salmon with a touch of spicy tomato sauce and guacamole, and asparagus with mustardy-mayonnaise**. There is just something about roasted asparagus covered in mayonnaise and a squeeze of lemon that is undeniably delicious. Fish two or three times a week is a good goal, and it's smart to keep salmon, a fattier fish, in heavy rotation.

2. **Steak and avocado with a side of sautéed spinach**. Need I say more?

3. **A magnificent salad filled with low-carb, high-fat goodies**. Start with two cups of arugula or spinach leaves as the base, add some thinly chopped red cabbage for color and crunch, throw in a whole avocado, include some chicken, tuna, or sardines for protein and a handful of sliced olives for a salty accent. Finish with a sprinkle of sesame, sunflower, or hemps seeds and some freshly grated sharp cheese (cheddar or Parmesan are fantastic), and top with sea salt, fresh ground pepper, and a homemade vinaigrette. I feed this to friends who think salad is "boring" and they are quickly transported to a happy place. The word "salad" is actually code for "leaves with good stuff on top." The ketogenic diet gives you license to go crazy on the fat-rich toppings. Be creative!

4. **Chicken with Cauliflower Mashed Potatoes.** For the chicken, sauté with olive oil, tamari, a squeeze of lemon juice, smoked paprika, and a dash of cayenne pepper, and Cauliflower Mashed Potatoes (page 272) on the side.

5. **Kelp noodles and tofu strips with basil pesto and a bowl of cream of mushroom soup**. This meal may seem like it's on the lighter side, but the cream in the soup and the oil in the pesto are quite filling. I like to use homemade beef broth for the soup, and that, together with the mushrooms, gives an intense umami flavor that is super satisfying. You can use tofu noodles in place of kelp noodles for a slightly heavier dish, but really it's the pesto that makes it special.

6. **Spice-rubbed pork chops and broccoli cooked in coconut oil**. If you've never made a meat rub, now is your chance to give it a shot. Mix together a bunch of dry spices in a bowl (cumin and paprika are common) and sprinkle the stuff all over a pork chop before you sear it in a very hot pan on both sides and then finish in a hot oven. The Broccoli in Coconut Oil recipe is on page 277.

I'll Have the One with Fewer Carbs, Thanks!

One of the most common mistakes on the ketogenic diet is not accurately accounting for the carbs in vegetables and nuts. These foods are an important part of a healthy diet, and you should be eating them. But pay attention to the carb count, and choose wisely. Similar foods are not all created equal. Take leafy greens, for example: Two cups of shredded romaine lettuce (about the amount in a small salad) contains just 1 g of net carbs, but the same amount of shredded kale contains 7 g of net carbs. One quarter cup of walnuts contains about 2 g of net carbs. Almonds have slightly more, about 3 g per quarter cup. But the same amount of cashews contains 10 g of net carbs. It's easy to see how you can unknowingly go over your daily carb limit. Become familiar with the carb content of the foods you eat on a regular basis. If you don't have to waste a few grams per day on something that you could easily swap for a similar food, then don't!

Dispelling the Myth of "Dietary Boredom"

Some people think that because you will be eating only poultry, fish, meat, vegetables, dairy, nuts, and oils on the ketogenic diet, you will be bored with your food choices. But do not fool yourself into thinking it's the ketogenic diet that relegates you to this perceived "food boredom"! If you want to have any type of healthful diet—ketogenic or not—you will have to face the fact that there are only so many raw materials to work with.

Keeping Things Interesting

So, chicken it is. Again. Sound boring? Well let me ask you this: why do you think chicken tastes so much better at a restaurant? After all, chicken is chicken is chicken, whether you have rice alongside it or not. Why is it "boring" to eat chicken at home but all of a sudden exciting to eat it at a restaurant? The answer is that *restaurants use sauces and spices*. Chicken can be blackened, or sautéed with lemon and rosemary, or grilled with a cumin-chili-cilantro rub. Broccoli can have an Italian flair when prepared with olive oil, garlic, and hot red pepper; and you can give the same vegetable an Asian flavor by using sesame oil, ginger, garlic, and soy sauce. Same raw materials, totally different tastes. Culinary techniques, spices, and sauces give foods more exciting flavors. In Chapter 13: Recipes you will find some simple and quick sauces to make and keep on hand. Get in the habit of using these so that you can enjoy an infinite flavor palette despite using the same basic ingredients in your meals.

Spices pack flavor into a dish. They are usually helped by fat, which carries flavor—one of the reasons why fat is so important in cooking. If you fail to add spices to your dishes—keto or not—they will be bland. Have you ever used smoked paprika, turmeric, or espelette pepper? If you don't know your way at all around a kitchen I highly recommend you ask a friend who enjoys cooking to show you a few techniques for using spices and making sauces, or get yourself a basic kitchen technique cookbook and learn to make salad dressings, mayonnaise, and the like. You might also consider getting a cookbook catering to a very-low-carb diet (few books use the term "ketogenic"), or even the paleo diet, which will have a lot of recipes suitable for the ketogenic dieter.

Aside from sauces and spices, there are other aspects of cooking that keep things interesting. Balancing different tastes—sweet, salty, sour, bitter, umami—offer one layer of variety. Even though we minimize sugar in the ketogenic diet, there is a still an element of sweetness that comes in from vegetables, dairy, nuts, and other foods that have a bit of sugar, as well as alternative sweeteners (if you choose to use them). We have lots of room to play with other elements of food appeal, including aroma, visual appeal, and temperature. Don't underutilize these elements when creating your meals. Pay attention to texture. Fat is soft and smooth, protein is chewy, and vegetables are crunchy. Sprinkle sesame seeds on top of your chicken or put nuts in your salad, then cover with sauce or dressing, and you'll easily see how the textural interplay makes a more satisfying meal. Pair cool things with warm things, or red things with yellow and green things (and purple and orange things) and you'll find a universe of meal possibilities! Chapter 13 "Recipes" will get you started with some delicious ketogenic recipes.

CHAPTER 9

Eating Out

Call to memory the last meal you ate at a restaurant. Did it occur to you that there might have been flour in your steak sauce, or sugar in your salad dressing? Could you possibly have predicted that the "mixed vegetables" accompanying your chicken dish would include potatoes?

Dining out can be treacherous for anyone with dietary restrictions. It's simply impossible to figure out the ingredients in every unique dish just by reading the menu. The first rule is always: ask. Thanks to the growing awareness of food allergies and attention to dietary restrictions, restaurants are becoming more adept at modifying dishes to meet the specific food needs of individual customers. A growing number of establishments is offering gluten-free or vegan menus—a testament to the fact that kitchens can prepare many items without certain "standard" ingredients. Some places may not be willing or able to alter the food to your liking, but many others will do just what you ask. The important thing is—ask! Also, do some research before you dine, asking for a nutritional facts brochure on site, or visiting the restaurant website in advance.

Eat as You Wish

It's no question that you have less control over the ingredients in your food when you eat something you haven't prepared yourself. This is true of restaurant meals, dining at friends' homes, and eating something out of a box or package—and it's true whether or not you're on a diet or following a certain eating plan. Few people like everything prepared just the way it's offered in any given establishment. Aren't there some ingredients you just can't stand? How about onions? Mushrooms? Cilantro? Blue cheese? Just consider the simple example of a fruit salad: in all the years that you relied on fruit as your "healthy snack," did you ever get fruit salad prepared with all of your favorite fruit and none of the things you dislike? I would be surprised if you did. Have you ever noticed that fruit salad from a store or restaurant has too much melon and not enough berries? Would you make it that way at home?

Well, thankfully, we've moved on from fruit salad, both because it's never prepared to our liking, and because it never resolves our hunger (it's all sugar, after all)! But the poor little fruit salad serves as a great example to illustrate the point that, when eating out, sometimes you will encounter things *you don't want*. It doesn't really matter *why* you don't want them. *You don't have to justify your preferences to anyone.* In fact, I'm a big fan of blue cheese, and if you came to my house for dinner you'd probably find it in your salad! If you told me you didn't want any, it wouldn't occur to me to interrogate you as to why that was and persuade you to change your mind. That would seem rather intrusive and impolite. Your reasons for wanting to eat the foods you eat are your own, and no one else has greater authority to determine what gets down the hatch. You left that game behind when you were seven, and mom and dad had to force you to eat your green beans. You're a grown-up now; eat what you want and ignore others when they act as if they know what's better for you.

Where to Start

It goes without saying that bread, pasta, potatoes, and other starches and grains are an absolute no-nos when eating out on the ketogenic diet. That goes for desserts, too (although homemade low-carb desserts are very popular in the keto community, the restaurant industry hasn't yet caught on!).

Once you set aside all the sugary starchy things, you can see pretty easily that there are a lot of dining out options. Restaurants are great at the traditional meat-and-vegetable-with-a-sauce type of dish. The sauce is usually made with butter or some other fat because restaurants are not afraid to use fat in their cooking. Chefs know that fat carries flavor, and they use it liberally. (That's one of the reasons why everything tastes better at a restaurant.) Sometimes these typical dishes are meat, starch, and vegetable; that problem is easy enough to solve: ask them to hold the starch. If they won't, then just leave that part on your plate.

Tip

Ask if there is a low-carb or gluten-free menu, or menu items that can be identified as such. Although these dishes are not guaranteed to be fully keto-friendly, they are a very good place to start.

Become a Curious Diner

Restaurant foods are undoubtedly a source of hidden carbs, so you really have to be curious about the ingredients in your meals and get comfortable asking questions. Many sauces, for example, are thickened with flour or cornstarch, which are super-high-carb ingredients to be completely avoided on the ketogenic diet. But sauces can also be thickened with butter or heavy cream, both completely allowed on the ketogenic diet. Find out what's in sauces and in dishes in general, and ask for preparations that you can enjoy. (As an added bonus, when you begin to learn the ingredients in dishes and sauces you love, you can replicate them at home!)

Sugar That's Strayed Where It Shouldn't Have

Once you start asking for the ingredient lists you'll be surprised to learn all the things that have sugar in them. One of my favorite healthy grocers, which also has a thriving prepared foods business, sells a dish called Cilantro Pesto Tofu. Sounds harmless. But when I checked the ingredients it turned out they use this recipe for pesto:

Cilantro
Expeller-pressed non-GMO canola oil
Lime juice
Ginger
Garlic
Jalapeños
Beet sugar
Salt

Huh? I figured cilantro pesto would have different ingredients from basil pesto, which has olive oil, nuts, and Parmesan cheese. The combination of lime, jalapeño, and garlic with cilantro made sense, because the herb is commonly found with those ingredients in guacamole. But I certainly wasn't expecting the beet sugar! I ordered the dish anyway, because in the my entire meal I probably had two tablespoons of the pesto sauce and thus a very small amount of the sugar. But asking for the ingredients and knowing that I'd had some sugar in that meal helped me keep track of the rest of my carbs throughout the day.

Carbs can pop up in many unexpected places. Did you know that:

- Maple syrup is often used to sweeten bacon?
- Fish is often lightly floured before being sautéed?
- Protein items (meat, poultry, or fish) may be breaded, even if the menu doesn't mention breading?
- Marinades very commonly contain sugar, honey, or some other sweetener?
- Sweeteners and starches are commonly used in sausage, sliced meats, or charcuterie?

The Ever-Popular "Mixed Vegetables"

Whenever you see something labeled in a vague manner like this you have to ask what's in the mix. For example:

- **Vegetable frittata.** Which vegetables, exactly, are in the frittata?
- **Baked fish with roasted vegetables.** Again, which vegetables?
- **Crudités**. This is a fancy name for a platter of raw vegetables. It may very well be the perfect thing,

complete with cucumber sticks, endive, and a cheese accompaniment. But it *may* be half crackers and bread, and the other half carrots and blanched potatoes that you want to avoid.

Restaurants have their own way of preparing things, and just because something falls into the vegetable category doesn't mean it's okay for you to eat. Non-starchy vegetables only, and you have to ask to know what's coming.

Preparations of Meat, Poultry, and Fish

If you're eating meat at a restaurant it may very likely be covered in a sauce that contains sugar, starch, or flour. Ask the server for a simple "au jus" (liquid left in the pan from the meat itself), or tell them beforehand that you're unable to eat flour or sweeteners. Steak sauce commonly contains such thickeners. Pork or venison are often prepared with a fruit-based sauce such as apples or cherries. Don't assume that burgers or meatballs are carb-free; many recipes call for breadcrumbs. Surprisingly, even meats that are listed as baked or broiled on the menu will be topped with breadcrumbs. It's an awkward moment indeed when the meat dish arrives covered in bread, and you have to send it back. Even if a menu item seems carb-free, ask the server to describe the preparation. If they don't give you all the information, you may have to probe with questions like:

- Is the fish breaded?
- Is there any breading or flour in this dish at all?
- Do you use cornstarch? Flour? Sugar? Honey?
- Or simply say "I don't eat starch or sugar" to get the conversation rolling.

"Broiled," You Say?

In my second week on the ketogenic diet I was out to dinner with a friend at a cozy little restaurant. My friend ordered a grass-fed burger, and she thought I should get one, too (minus the bun) since the waiter said it was delicious. I was in the mood for something lighter, though, so I ordered the "Broiled pollock with asparagus and cauliflower." Great! Broiled fish with two servings of low-carb vegetables. A perfect keto meal.

But when my plate arrived, the fish was smothered in breadcrumbs. Apparently in this establishment, "broiled" meant "covered with breadcrumbs first, and then broiled." They'd forgotten to mention that first part in the description of the dish on the menu. I looked at my friend, and she looked at me, and we didn't know what to do. It was a small place, and I felt bad about returning the dish. I tried to pick at the fish underneath the topping, but there was absolutely no way to "eat around" a plateful of breadcrumbs. I had to return it. I told the waiter that I was sorry, but I was unable to eat the dish because of the breadcrumbs and that I really wished they'd have mentioned that on the menu, as the term "broiled" on its own does not usually imply "breaded" as well.

The waiter apologized for the miscommunication and exchanged my plate for a lovely, plain-broiled fish and vegetables. There would be many more restaurant trip-ups in my keto-dining days, but this was the first and it taught me a very important lesson: do not assume that a dish is what it says it is. *Always ask.*

The Customer Gets What the Customer Requests

Oftentimes a server being questioned about the ingredients in a dish will interrupt and ask "what are you allergic to?" They're trying to speed up the discussion by pinpointing what they believe will be the one ingredient you need to avoid, steering you toward a dish without that ingredient. This tactic can certainly work, but it's often not sufficient for the ketogenic dieter. Servers are usually surprised that in addition to, say, bread, you also choose to avoid rice, potatoes, and quinoa. Try to explain to the person that the number of things you're unwilling to eat is likely far greater than the number of ingredients in the dish you're considering ordering, and that it will be less time-consuming for them to give you information rather than the other way around.

Lest you worry about being a nag, let's clarify something straightaway: the bar and restaurant industry is also known as "the service industry." These establishment exist to serve you food and beverages to your satisfaction. If someone is making you feel rushed to order from a menu that doesn't provide you with the information you need, or you begin to feel guilty for taking too much of their time or asking too many questions, just take a deep breath, look the person calmly in the eye, and say, "I'm really looking forward to this meal, and I'm hoping you can help me get the information I need." Then, proceed with your questions. Saying in a calm tone something like, "I'm trying hard to take care of my health, and there are many things I can't eat. Forgive me for causing you inconvenience," will do a lot to get people on your side. It's easier to garner empathy by speaking from the heart than it is by being combative.

A small number of servers are very eager to respond to your requests and help you navigate the menu. These personalities will be interested in what you're doing and may ask questions out of their own curiosity. You can share your eating parameters with these folks and ask them to help you explore the menu for appropriate items. They'll know what can be modified (for example, leaving off a sauce that contains cornstarch) and what cannot (for example, chicken fillets that have already been dredged in flour). And, in turn, you'll be educating them on the ketogenic diet. Consider it an exchange!

Restaurants will often accommodate changes to dishes that don't require extra work or ingredients. If you're asking for something more expensive than what's listed on the menu, then you may have to be willing to pay an extra buck or two for the higher-quality ingredient. For example, if you order a burger (hold the bun) that comes with fries, but you want a green salad or side of sautéed spinach instead, keep in mind that spinach and salad are more nutritious than potatoes, and they cost more, too.

If you just want them to leave something off (for example, leaving off the croutons on a salad, or putting the dressing on the side) then they should be able to do that with no argument and certainly for no extra charge.

Restaurants that insist that they can't make modifications at all, even to leave off ingredients, are just really committed to their menu and their way of doing things, and it's not worth battling. Find something on their menu that suits you, or find other businesses to patronize.

Many places *will* accommodate, especially in today's food and health environment where food allergies and diet restrictions are common. Some customers could have life-threatening allergic reactions if a peanut sauce or oil so much as touched their plate. These people safeguard their health with confidence by asking about ingredients, despite the potential for irritating some impatient servers. Follow their lead and don't be shy. Ask for what you need. Restaurants don't want angry customers on their hands (let alone a pair of paramedics in their dining room!).

Is That Not What You Ordered?

Often a server will check an ingredient list with the kitchen, you'll approve the dish, and it will come out with items that weren't mentioned. One day while I was keto dieting I ordered brunch at a café. On the menu was a Farmers' Market Vegetable Frittata. I asked which vegetables were in the frittata. The server didn't know, so he went to the kitchen to inquire and returned to announce the mix: asparagus, tomatoes, broccoli, and artichokes. Great! Could I get it without the artichokes and the potatoes that came on the side? We had a back and forth about my dietary preferences, and it was decided that I could.

When the dish came out it contained *none* of the vegetables mentioned. Instead, there were carrots, mushrooms, and zucchini. The server came to ask me how my dish was. I spoke up. "Well, you told me there would be asparagus, tomatoes, and broccoli in here and actually there are carrots, mushrooms, and zucchini."

"Well, the chef just puts a mix of whatever he has in the back."

"Ah, is that so? I'm struggling to understand…given that we had such a long conversation about it, and you actually went to the kitchen to ask what was in the dish, how it could be that the dish arrived with a completely different set of ingredients? Some people are highly allergic to mushrooms, you know."

"Do you want me to replace it?"

"Well do you actually *have* the dish you mentioned? Because it sounded good to me."

"I'll check."

The waiter returned with an asparagus, tomato, and broccoli frittata.

I felt a little bad for being so pushy, but it also felt good to hold him accountable. I wasn't even so put out in the carb sense; I could have eaten around the carrots in the other dish and stayed within my carb allotment. But I was really annoyed that I'd been offered one thing and served another. If, when the check came out to $13 I chose to pay only $9, I don't think the waiter would have been very pleased. The menu is the start of a contract between the diner and the establishment; by ordering, you are agreeing to pay after you've eaten as long as the item comes out as described. If not, all bets are off.

Had I not spoken up to the waiter that day I'd have been annoyed, frustrated that I ate more carbs than I wanted to (I might have snuck a few bites of carrot, you never know), and feeling like the universe had undermined my efforts to stay on track. Don't sit back and let yourself fall into a victim mentality, using that to say that dieting is too hard and you're no good at it. Ask for what you need, and you will often get it.

General Guidelines for Eating Out Low-Carb

You won't always have the opportunity to get a food prepared exactly to your ideal specifications, so you may have to make *small* compromises. *This doesn't mean that you should simply eat whatever is offered if it doesn't meet your standards.* Not at all! But perhaps you can spare the few carbs in a steak marinade made with brown sugar while having dinner at a restaurant, and forego the strawberries you were planning to eat at home later on. Remember that while it's important to know which foods contain carbs, you don't have to be an absolute maniac about keeping every carb out of your mouth! Some foods contain just a very small amount, and adjusting your carb intake elsewhere in the day may give you much greater freedom to enjoy meals eaten out.

Knowing how to choose low-carb restaurant dishes and avoid common "dining out" pitfalls will quell your anxiety about going out to eat. Here are some guidelines for finding appropriate meals at a variety of restaurants serving different types of cuisine.

Bar/Pub-Style Restaurant

I don't recommend eating at places whose main business activity is serving alcohol. The quality of food tends to be lower, and the menus may be limited to only a few items. It can be a challenge to get a keto meal in a place like this.

That said, if you need to eat at a bar or pub, here are some basic tips that will help get you through:

Know Before You Go

In addition to the resources in the back of the book, these sites are particularly helpful in learning tricks for dining out low-carb:

- The Atkins Foundation also has a useful section on dining out while on the Atkins diet, which begins as a ketogenic diet. Keep in mind that the Atkins diet starts out very strict, with only 12–15 g of carbs allowed per day, and becomes more lenient over time. www.atkins.com

- The Celiac Disease Foundation has a Dining Out Guide with suggestions for avoiding gluten that may prevent you from accidentally consuming hidden carbohydrates from bread and wheat products. It won't alert you to hidden sources of starch or sugar from non-wheat foods, and, remember—because not all sources of gluten contain carbohydrates, some of the foods they recommend avoiding (e.g., soy sauce), are okay for you to eat. But because wheat is such a widely used food ingredient in restaurant dishes, and because these dishes often do contain carbohydrate, this guide is a very good reference. http://celiac.org

- Have a burger and skip the bun.
- Have mayonnaise and mustard, but no ketchup.
- If they have only fried proteins, like chicken fingers or fried fish, scrape off the breading.
- Ask for salad dressing *on the side*; the dressing is probably not made in-house and likely to have sweeteners and starches.

- Ask if they have a breakfast menu, and if so, see if you can order off of that. Bars and pubs tend to have steak-and-egg type breakfasts, or omelets.
- Ask if meat patties contain breadcrumbs, and if so, order something else.
- Avoid veggie burgers, which are typically patties of grains and legumes.

Café/Coffee Shop

It can be super easy or terribly difficult to eat keto in a café or coffee shop, depending on their menu. Some cafés are full-blown restaurants, while others have just a pastry case and a coffee counter. It's usually hard to tell which type it is from the outside, so it's worth going in to have a peek around.

Tips for eating at a café or coffee shop:

- Obviously, avoid all pastries and breads—even those that are gluten-free! Gluten-free does not mean carb-free.
- If you are confronted with a pastry counter and nothing else, look carefully to see if you can find a basket of boiled eggs. You will probably find one half the time.
- If it's morning, ask if they have a lunch menu. Some cafés are small enough that they only display lunch foods when lunch rolls around. They may have sandwiches that you can eat sans bread, or, if you're lucky, a salad or two.
- If all else fails, eat the eggy inside of a piece of quiche. Leave the crust.

- Ordering coffee: Almost every coffee shop will have alternative sweetener. But be careful—some of the sugar packets look like alternative sweetener packets, and you don't want to dump a load of sugar in your coffee. If you like it milky, most places have half-and-half, and many have heavy cream, although it's rarely placed out for customers' use. Ask.

To Coffee or Not to Coffee?

Coffee has no carbs. It does have antioxidant compounds that have been shown to have various health-promoting effects, including preventing dementia and heart disease. But let's face it: most of us drink coffee for the kick, not for its healthfulness. Caffeine is what's called an "ergogenic aid": it increases alertness and energy level, suppresses appetite, and can temporarily increase blood pressure and heart rate. The vast majority of research on the effects of caffeine on human functioning is done by the US military (since those folks may often need to perform well on little sleep). It's a valuable tool for getting through mental sluggishness and bodily fatigue, and it works best when not overused. Studies show that if you take breaks from caffeine use it will work better when you use it again. There's no formal "upper limit" set for caffeine but, 400 mg per day, or about four cups of coffee or green tea, is generally considered the safe maximum.

There is no restriction for coffee on the ketogenic diet, but it is important to watch your caffeine intake and monitor how you feel. Some people have trouble with caffeine on the diet because of changes in hydration status or blood sugar. It's a smart idea to observe your physical symptoms and set limits for yourself that keep you feeling well.

There *is* a restriction on the variety of sweeteners and "fluff" people add to their coffee. It probably doesn't need to be said that you should stay away from mochaccinos and other "blended" or sweetened coffee beverages. There are too many varieties of these to list, so, if it tastes like a coffee milkshake, just say no! Keep it simple. Stick to black coffee, to which you can add alternative sweetener if you'd like without jeopardizing ketosis. Heavy cream, which has zero carbs, is also on the "okay" list. Half-and-half is closer to whole milk, and each of these has about 1.5 g of carbs per fluid ounce. Since that's about how much you'll use in your coffee, you may be able to get away with that once or twice a day if that's how you want to use your carb allotment.

Chinese

Chinese food is probably the worst culprit when it comes to hidden carbs. We already know that sauces contain sugars and starches, and that rice and noodles are common. Cornstarch can easily lurk in soups, or as a light coating for meats and vegetables before they are stir-fried.

Tips for eating at a Chinese restaurant:

- Almost all sauces contain carbs. Ask for meals without sauce, and use soy sauce for flavor.
- Beef, chicken, or tofu entrees with vegetables are a safe bet (without sauce). Whole fish is another good option.
- Ask for vegetables steamed instead of in garlic sauce.
- Order clear broth soups, and ask if they contain any thickeners.
- Avoid mixed vegetables, which often contain corn and carrots. Ask for Chinese greens instead.

Bread Goes by Many Names

There is almost an endless variety of foods that use bread, breadcrumbs, or wheat flour to some extent. While bread and pasta are obviously made of flour, some other terms might not be so familiar. Avoid any of the following items:

- Pain
- Pan
- Challah
- Brioche
- Sourdough
- Baguette
- Panko
- Semolina
- Crust
- Pastry
- Pie
- Dough
- Muffin
- Scone
- Danish
- Cake
- Loaf
- Phyllo
- Filo

- Pita
- Panini
- Naan
- Injera
- Farina
- Dumpling
- Empanada
- Shumai
- Croissant
- Biscuit
- Crouton
- Kibbeh
- Couscous
- Tabbouleh
- Stroganoff
- Napoleon
- Mille-feuille
- Wonton

French

It's easy to get a keto meal at a French restaurant. The French love fat, especially in the form of butter and cheese. They're not afraid of bread or sugar, though, so be careful to avoid those ingredients.

Tips for eating keto at a French restaurant:

- Tartares are very popular, especially steak or tuna. It's unusual to eat without bread, but you can certainly do it! The steak will come with mustard and small pickles called *cornichon*, which are keto friendly.

- Starter salads are usually a safe bet. Frisee with *lardons* (pieces of pork fat similar to bacon) is a nice fatty option. A *nicoise* salad is made with salad greens, hard-boiled egg, green beans, tomatoes, tuna, and olives, as well as boiled potatoes. (Ask to leave the potatoes off.) A goat cheese salad is often made with the cheese on *croûte*, or big pieces of hard toast. Ask if you can have the cheese without the bread. If they tell you the cheese is melted onto the bread, ask if you can have unmelted cheese! Let's find a solution, people!

- Entrees are pretty easy at a French restaurant. Steak, chicken, or fish are often served with vegetables, usually cooked in butter, as well as a sauce, usually made with butter and flour. Politely ask if the kitchen can thicken the sauce with butter or cream instead. The French are fond of both. Rice or potatoes are often served on the side. Leave them aside or ask for none.

- A side of non-starchy vegetables, such as broccoli and cauliflower, or spinach sautéed in butter or olive oil, should be easy to come by. Sautéed mixed mushrooms with herbs may be a possibility.

- Breakfasts are also easy in French-leaning establishments. Egg omelets are ubiquitous, they come with vegetables, cheese, ham, or fine herbs and are often accompanied by a side salad and potatoes or bread. Skip the last two. Poached eggs are another common French breakfast. Some establishments will have fromage blanc, a yogurt-like cheese that is usually carb-free. It's almost always served with fruit. Just order it plain.

- The fun thing about dining keto at a French restaurant is that the French believe wholly in cheese for dessert, and they make some of the best cheeses! If you're out with friends eating chocolate mousse or apple tarts and you're feeling deprived, order a cheese plate. You will of course leave the bread untouched.

Italian

Don't be fooled into thinking you can't eat at an Italian restaurant—they serve much more than just pasta! Most Italian menus are separated into appetizers/salads, pasta (*primi*), and protein-based entrees (*secondi*). You can find many things to eat.

Tips for eating at an Italian restaurant:

- Peruse the salad options, as there will likely be something that fits your needs. Many Italian restaurants use sweet balsamic vinegars, so ask if you can swap for red wine vinegar instead.

- Grilled vegetable platters may be an option, but these may include some starchier vegetables, so you will want to ask for details.

- Many meat or chicken dishes are breaded. If you don't understand the menu description (such as Milanese or Piccata), ask how it's prepared. There will almost always be options for plain chicken, meat, or fish with a light sauce.

- Tomato sauce is usually a source of some carbs. A pomodoro sauce is better than a marinara sauce. Pesto is a good choice. Cream sauces may or may not have carbs—you must ask.

Sugar and Starch in Cured Meats

A ketogenic dieter will notice that one of the "safest" appetizers on any restaurant menu is the charcuterie plate: a variety of meats, perhaps with some cheeses and olives (hold the bread), and you're good to go. Unfortunately, these meats are not always carb-free. Sugar is used widely in the curing of meats and dry sausages to help retain flavor and red color. Starches and flours are used to keep in moisture and to help bind the fat and protein components. Many restaurants make their own cured meats, so it's often easy to find out what's in them. Ask your server; if they don't cure items in-house, they may still know the basics of what's sweet and what's not. As always, just ask.

Japanese

Japanese food highlights fish and sea vegetables, both of which are great keto options, and most menus also have meat (okay), starchy vegetables (not okay), and of course, rice (definitely not okay). Sake is wine made from rice that will vary in carb content, but you can generally estimate 1.5 g carbs per ounce of sake.

Tips for eating at a Japanese restaurant:

- Order sashimi instead of sushi, so you get just the fish without the rice. The vinegar used on the fish is usually sweetened, so ask for the fish plain or just account for a couple of grams of carbs.

- Some places will accommodate a request for sushi rolls without the rice, so that it's just fish or vegetable wrapped in nori (seaweed), which is perfectly keto-friendly. If you don't like nori it may be possible to have your fish wrapped in very thinly sliced cucumber, or a soy wrapper, which should be carb-free or close to it. Be very careful with sauces brushed onto the rolls or in fish that's chopped and prepared with some other ingredients, as these will almost always contain sweeteners.

- Make sure that your items don't come with "crunch" or panko, which are Japanese breadcrumbs.

- Check the "yakitori" menu section, which usually lists grilled meats and vegetables on skewers. Japanese meat preparations tend to have sweetened sauces (such as teriyaki sauce), so inquire about the marinades or ask for the meat plain and have an unsweetened sauce (such as soy sauce) on the side.

- Teriyaki and other sauces may be thickened with starch even if they don't contain sugar. If your dish comes with something the consistency of barbecue sauce, be wary.

- Clear soups like miso should be a safe choice. Miso soup is a clear broth with a small bit of tofu and some seaweed. It should have little to no carbs.

- Fresh green salads are on most menus, but the dressing will very likely be sweet. Carrot-ginger or miso-ginger are likely culprits. Ask if they have another option for dressing that doesn't contain sugar, or ask for it on the side and use very sparingly. The same is true of seaweed or cucumber salad; these most likely contain sugar, so account for a gram or two in your carb allotment if you eat them.

- Starchy vegetables are very popular in Japanese cuisine. Items like mountain yam and burdock root are just as carb-heavy as potatoes and corn, and should be avoided. It's hard to identify whether vegetables are starchy or not from their names on menus. If you see something unfamiliar, ask the server to describe what it is.

- Beware of "imitation" crab meat. This is not crab but surimi, a fish paste made of inexpensive white fish mixed with sugar, wheat flour, fish flavorings, and preservatives. In grocery stores it is labeled as imitation crab, but restaurant menus can obscure the true nature of this product. Sometimes called "crab sticks" or "fish cake," it's often found inside the California roll, or in ramen or other Japanese soups. It's used as a cheaper ingredient in things like seafood salad. You can tell surimi from real fish by the taste and texture: it is somewhat rubbery and stringy, has a bit of a sweet flavor, and it will have a streak of bright, reddish-orange in its mostly white "flesh."

Mexican

Mexican restaurants tend to organize their menus around the various types of tortilla-filled items known commonly to the American diner: tacos, burritos, enchiladas, and fajitas. Pretty much everything is served with rice and beans, and chips and salsa are always within reach.

Given the preponderance of starch-based foods at most Mexican restaurants, they can be an intimidating place to try to get a keto meal. But that's a superficial view! Once you take a deeper look you'll notice that Mexican restaurants are pretty friendly to the ketogenic dieter.

Tips for eating at a Mexican restaurant:

- Check out the true entrees section. Mexican food is not just tacos and burritos! Entrees are generally similar to those in other restaurants, just prepared with different flavors. Steak, chicken, and fish dishes are very common. Sauces are usually tomato or broth-based (rather than flour-based), which is a positive.

- Most plates are served with rice and beans, and you can skip those.

- Fajitas are a very good bet. They usually come with grilled meat, chicken, fish, or tofu and vegetables. You'll certainly be leaving the tortillas on the side.

- Guacamole and sour cream are okay to eat. Watch out for guacamoles that have fruit, like pineapple or mango versions.

- Salsas usually have some sweetener, so ask for a fresh pico de gallo, which is generally the same ingredients (tomatoes and onion), without sugar.

- Mexican salads often contain jicama and mango. Jicama is okay in small amounts. Mango should be avoided. Ask them to leave it off.

- If tacos and burritos are the only thing on the menu, eat the good stuff on the inside and leave behind the bready exterior (as usual).

Hidden Sources of Fruits

Restaurants love to make use of dried, sugared, or stewed fruits to lend a sweet flavor to savory dishes. These are concentrated sources of sugar and should not be eaten, even if you are moving into the lenient phases of your diet. Look out for the following:

- Salads prepared at restaurants are a likely source of dried fruit, especially raisins, dried cranberries, and dates.

- Pork and duck dishes are often paired with fruit compotes made of apple, cherry, orange, and the like. If you're not sure what's in the sauce from reading the menu, ask.

- Cheese or meat (charcuterie) platters often come with some sort of jam or jelly. In Spanish restaurants you may see the term "quince paste," a sort of jelly made from the very sweet quince fruit. As with other jellies, this food is very high in sugar and should not be eaten, even in small amounts.

Middle Eastern

Middle Eastern restaurants are pretty easy places to eat keto meals.

Tips for eating at a Middle Eastern restaurant:

- Meat, chicken, or shrimp skewers are a good choice. They are often served with a lot of rice, which you can give to a friend.

- Order a typical diced cucumber and tomato salad, which will be dressed with lemon juice and olive oil.

- Try a small portion of baba ghanoush, which is dip made of eggplant that's lower in carbs than hummus (made of chickpeas). These two are likely to be on every menu. Ask for cucumber sticks to eat these with, instead of pita bread.

- Ask for tahini, which is a delicious creamy sauce made of ground sesame seeds, as a high-fat, low-carb topping for anything.

- Lamb or chicken shawarma (meats roasted on a spit and sliced), are often served as sandwiches along with lettuce, cucumbers, tomatoes, and some dressing. Order and consume these carefully: make sure the dressing is not carb-heavy, and eat just the fillings from inside the pita, leaving the bread behind.

- There are some fantastic spices used in Middle Eastern cuisine that we don't see elsewhere. Z'aatar is a mix of green herbs and sesame seeds that comes often on bread; sumac looks like red pepper but tastes like lemon. You can ask for sides of these to flavor your food.

- Avoid tabbouleh, a salad made with couscous (a grain), and kibbeh, which are meatballs made with bulgur (also a grain).

Sauces to Avoid

Unless you know the ingredients in the particular preparation being offered to you, avoid the following sauces:

- White sauce
- Brown sauce
- Gravy
- Roux
- Glaze (or glazed)
- Sweet-and-sour sauce
- Barbecue sauce
- Garlic sauce
- Stir-fry sauce
- Teriyaki sauce
- Cheese sauce
- Cream sauce
- Orange sauce
- Asian marinade
- Duck sauce
- Hoisin sauce
- Mole
- Steak sauce
- Dipping sauce
- Peanut sauce
- Chutney

Salad Bar

Salad bars are *usually* great! Here, you can pick your own fixings from individual items, so you won't have to worry much about inadvertent carb contamination. Still, carbs can lurk in unforeseen places, so here are some general tips.

- Start with a nice base of salad greens like spinach, romaine lettuce, or arugula; add in protein like shredded chicken, tuna, or cubed tofu; add some olives, cucumbers, and other vegetables.
- Avoid any protein items that look like they have a brown sauce (e.g., barbecue chicken, tofu in garlic sauce).

- Watch out for shredded cheeses, which can contain additives that might have carbohydrates. Choose the cheese that is labeled as a type, such as Parmesan, blue, or Swiss, rather than just "shredded cheese."
- Don't use salad dressing in a bottle, especially low-fat or fat-free dressings. A proper fat-rich dressing contains oil and vinegar or another acidic ingredient (such as lemon), and these are emulsified by whisking, blending, or by the addition of another item that contains fat, such as egg or cream. Fat-free salad dressings, since they can't use oil, rely on other thickening and emulsifying ingredients like, you guessed it—sugars and starches. If oil and vinegar are not provided at the salad bar ask an employee to get you some. Often they are willing to whisk the two together for you to get a thicker consistency, and you can put that on your salad. Choose red wine or white wine vinegar instead of balsamic, which has more carbs per serving.

CHAPTER 10

Tips for Making the Ketogenic Diet Work

Successful dieting requires continuous motivation from a variety of sources both internal and external. Here are twenty-six ways to make sure the ketogenic diet works for you!

Set reminders on your phone or computer that encourage you throughout the week.

What's the one thing you need to hear when you're feeling discouraged or feel like giving up? Is it a straightforward positive cheer, like, "Hey there, you can do it!" Or something profound that acknowledges your struggle, like, "The only way *out* is *through*." Perhaps you need frequent reminders to "ask what's in the sauce" or a panic-button sort of calendar pop-up that says "remember the stevia-sweetened chocolate bar is in the freezer for emergencies only." If you take only one suggestion from this section, take this one: YOU are your own best guide, and YOU know best what you need. Be a support for your future self by anticipating your needs and setting multiple reminders like these. You will be amazed at how frequently they pop up just when you need them.

Tap into the ocean of motivation in social media.

There is an endless supply of inspiring quotes, pictures of healthy dinner plates, ad hoc recipes, and before-and-after selfies of successful dieters in bikinis out there. It only takes a few of these each day to help you keep your eye on the prize. Search Facebook, Instagram, Tumblr, Pinterest, and other social media sites for terms like "diet motivation," "healthy eating," and "successful living." "Follow" or "Like" the pages of those who inspire you, and let them help usher you toward your goal. Even strategies for success that are unrelated to dieting can help you stay motivated. Keep looking for these, whether you do the diet for three months or as a long-term lifestyle.

Acknowledge your power to change.

Change is a process that requires active participation from you, the change agent. Think that's not you? Allow me to refresh your memory. Have you ever quit smoking? Given up a food you were allergic to? Have you ever started a new job, or gone to school, or moved to another house, or another city, or had kids? All of these things require motivation, critical thinking, action, and follow-through. You have made hundreds of changes in your life, many of which were probably not very easy. Don't sell yourself short. You are completely capable of making the changes you desire to live the life you want.

Come to terms with the fact that sugar and starch are making you overweight and sick.

You can do this now, or you can do it after you get diabetes. On the way to diabetes, your body cells become "insulin resistant," meaning that they don't respond to insulin's signal to let the sugar inside to be used for energy. Insulin, if you recall, tells your body to store fat. If you're trying to lose weight you don't want too much of it hanging around. But when you don't respond well to insulin the body produces more and more of it to force sugar into the cells against their resistance, and fatter and fatter you become. Insulin resistance is an enemy to fat loss, not to mention longevity and health. But you can absolutely prevent it by losing weight, changing your diet, and exercising. If you wait until you are diabetic to do these things then you won't be able to have the occasional indulgence of ice cream or birthday cake without also shooting yourself full of insulin. Sure makes option #1 look appealing, huh?

Make a formal commitment to someone you wouldn't want to let down.

We all have people in our lives to whom we look up, and whom we want to make proud. Think of someone like this in your life. They can be a dear friend, teacher, sibling, parent, child, etc. Pick someone who is willing and able to hear what's going on with you. You should be able to contact this person on a semi-regular basis, say, three to four times a month. Ask that person if they would be willing to hear your commitment to the ketogenic diet and hold you accountable. If they agree, make the commitment to them out loud or in writing. Be specific: say what the diet entails, how long you will do it, how much weight you want to lose, etc.

Explore your local grocery or health food store to hunt down low-carb foods.

Believe it or not, there is such a thing as carb-free bread. There are crackers and tomato sauces with less than 2 g of net carbs per serving. There are noodles made of kelp that have neither carbs nor calories. If you're not a food geek, you probably don't know that these things exist. They will help you not only to drop the weight while on keto, but also to stay slim and healthy over the long-term. Especially thanks to the paleo trend, food manufacturers are catering to the super-low-carb needs of consumers. The novel carb-free and low-carb foods mentioned throughout this book are items I've found both online and in my local grocery. Visit yours to see what's available. If you don't find much, consider talking to the purchasing manager to request items you'd like them to carry.

Start shopping at the farmers' market.

Going to a good farmers' market for your groceries is like having your personal dietitian pre-select the foods in the grocery store that you might actually want to eat, while leaving out the junk. Here you will find a beautiful bounty of fresh, whole foods that are perfect for the ketogenic diet! No boxed or packaged starchy or sugary foods at the farmers' market. Instead you'll see grass-fed beef and butter, pasture-raised chicken and eggs, organic non-starchy vegetables, locally caught fish, and the occasional appearance of perfectly sweet summer strawberries. If you're on the West Coast you can also get ripe avocados. Stay away from tubers and homemade baked goods.

Get excited about new flavors and cultivate a sense of adventure!

Are you the kind of person who needs to eat the same type of snack (usually sugary) every day around 4 p.m.? Must you have two cups of coffee before you leave the house? Do you eat a substantial meal for dinner, even on days when you're not that hungry? How is this routine working out for you? Did it ever occur to you that this might be a little... *boring*?

We hear so much criticism of diets for being restrictive and taking away freedom of choice, but we rarely notice the eating ruts we're in to start with. In my experience on the ketogenic diet I found that taking away foods I ate every day, such as yogurt, apples, and sweet potatoes, created space in my diet for new foods that had never before gotten much of my attention—things like coconut oil, sunflower seed butter, and seaweed snacks, interesting meats like venison and buffalo, and new spices and sauces. One of the best things about removing common foods from your diet is that you get the opportunity to try entirely new foods!

Check out ethnic grocery stores.

There are foods free of carbs (and those full of carbs) that you've never even heard of sold within a few miles of your home or workplace. While the US has spent the last fifty or so years trying to figure out how to get wheat and sugar into every imaginable food, other countries have continued to eat traditional cuisines based on a variety of healthful, whole foods. Most ethnic groceries will have a variety of foods that are suitable for the ketogenic dieter. Check out the Japanese grocery store for interesting produce like spiky cucumbers and shiso leaves. Most Mexican groceries will stock fresh salsas, as well as avocados and jalapeños for guacamole. Italian specialty stores will have cured meats, cheeses, and jarred items like olive tapenades. Search the Middle Eastern market for flavorful red pepper spread, jarred okra with tomato and onion, or fantastically wonderful spices like z'ataar, sumac, and aleppo, and stop at the deli counter for some *lebneh*, a type of yogurt-cheese that's very low in carbs. The possibilities are endless. Go explore! Just *be sure to read the labels!*

If it looks like a duck and quacks like a duck…

If you find yourself devouring some unfamiliar food with gusto, do a reality check on your carb-o-meter. Don't fool yourself into thinking that the dehydrated turnip chips you can't seem to stop eating are carb-free because they're not made of potatoes, or that the almond butter from an unlabeled container that tastes just a *little* too sweet doesn't contain sugar. Although there are some items like these that are absolutely keto-friendly (e.g., cauliflower chips, unsweetened almond butter), many products are like wolves in sheep's clothing. If you're having a cheat moment, okay, you're human; get back on board for dinner. But don't go about your day in willful denial. If it's dry and starchy-sweet, it's probably not something you want to eat.

Don't allow yourself to feel trapped by the amount of carbs in "one serving."

Be creative with your carb allotment! You're allowed to have one teaspoonful of something if one tablespoon has too many carbs. You can mix half a container of one thing with half a container of something else. It's really up to you! Whip out those multiplication and division skills from grade school and figure out what fits into your carb allotment for the day. This approach will give you much more freedom in your choice of foods and will help you sustain the ketogenic diet over the long term.

Learn to tell when you're hungry for food, hungry for something else, and when you're full.

The ketogenic diet works in part by taking away your feeling of hunger. If you insist on eating *regardless* of hunger then you may not lose the weight you want to lose. Learn how to tell when you're actually hungry, and when the "empty" feeling in your belly is really a cry for some other kind of nourishment. If you're familiar with the latter, you're not alone! We all have a need for different kinds of nurturing throughout our lives. When you're bored, find some form of amusement other than eating. When you're feeling scared or lonely, call up a friend or loved one instead of turning to food.

On a similar note, you risk staying at the same weight if you consistently eat bigger portions than you need. Learn how to tell when you are about 80 percent full, and prepare to take your last couple of bites. Do not continue eating once you are full. Ketogenic meals are very satisfying, and if you're the kind of person who usually eats with no end to your appetite (and this frustrates you), then you may be pleasantly surprised with your experience on the ketogenic diet.

Keep in mind that you will need less food on the ketogenic diet than you normally eat. It's unusual to "graze" all day, or to never quite feel full. If you find yourself eating more than three meals a day, or if your portion sizes are very large, then you may be overeating.

Write a "break up" letter with your favorite carb-heavy food.

We have almost all had the experience of breaking up with a significant other. It's usually a painful process in the beginning, and we'll do or say anything to avoid the inevitable split. Then, after the initial shock, we start to see all the positives about being without the other person. New experiences delight us, and we realize we've been "missing out." We wonder how we ever could have thought that it would be impossible to live without him/her! These shifting feelings are a sign that we've accepted a loss and have opened ourselves up to something new. You'll likely feel a similar grief at "losing" some foods that have long been a part of your life. So don't wait to be dumped! Instead, write a break up letter to the one food you know you're going to kick and scream before you give up. "Dear Pasta, I have to say goodbye now. I'm going to miss you terribly at first, but we both know it's for the best..."

Learn to take your coffee black.

Literally and figuratively. If there is something that you do *every day* that has you consuming sugar or starch, you've got to change that habit if you want to succeed on the ketogenic diet. If you have had tea with honey and toast or Cheerios every morning for breakfast for the last thirty years, then begin to try alternative sweeteners or tea with cream and eggs for breakfast. It may not be easy at first, but you will find it gets easier over time. If the thought of this makes you cringe, and if you have real concerns that this will derail your diet efforts, then begin to slowly wean yourself off of these things until you feel you are ready to take the leap, and then start the ketogenic diet.

Sugar is so ubiquitous in our foods that it's almost as if our taste buds have been hijacked for the sweet taste alone. Once you remove the sweet you'll notice a whole new world of fascinating flavors pop out at you. The major ones are sour, salty, bitter, and umami, but there are nuances like spicy, earthy, herbal, smoky, and an endless array of wonderfully delicious flavors our tongues were built to discern. Too bad for our non-keto friends whose taste buds continue to be assaulted by sugar: they're being robbed of the fascinating world of the savory. (Psst: If you're feeling benevolent, you might invite them to join us.)

Decide that it's okay to be hungry if you're stuck in a keto-unfriendly environment.

Let me reiterate: You will seldom be hungry on the ketogenic diet, and you'll be able to find something suitable to eat in most places. But in the unlikely event that you find yourself feeling peckish at an all-day bread-and-beer festival, just make the decision to accept your hunger. It will soon pass, and you will feel empowered having endured it. Dieting or not, the vast majority of us don't ever have the opportunity to stare down hunger. We move to feed our bellies as soon as we feel the tiniest grumble. Are you really that fragile? You weren't always that way. Remember when you were a kid in elementary school, and sometimes you got hungry a couple of hours before it was time for lunch? You just sat with your hunger and the world did not come to an end. You can do that now, too. Your other choice in this scenario would be to bulk up on bread and derail your diet. It's probably not worth it.

Prepare some go-to foods and beverages to keep around at all times.

Some of my clients make flavored drinks by putting a cinnamon stick or some mint leaves and strawberry slices in a jar of water to carry with them throughout the day. Some people swear by keto-baked goods made with erythritol and stevia, and keep these on hand at home or in the office. Others (myself included) are lost without a bag of almonds stashed strategically in the three places they spend the most time (e.g., home, work, car). The "Incredible Edible Egg" packs a good deal of nutrition into a low-calorie package. Eggs are satisfying and nutritious, cook in a flash, and can easily be carried for a snack later in the day. You can boil a few at a time to store, and easily grab some for breakfast or a snack when running out the door. We all have busy lives, and sooner or later you will be pressed for time and wanting a bite to eat. Don't let yourself be caught without appropriate food and tempted to eat something that will blow your diet. Prepare in advance.

Remake your kitchen into a no-carb space.

Why not make it easy on yourself? Completely remove things that would temp you to fall off the wagon, like crackers, jams, and other shelf-stable, starchy goodies hiding in the cabinet. Once you've done that, take a closer look and see what is just a bit too high in carbs to be a good companion for you as a ketogenic dieter. Start by reading the labels on the containers in your refrigerator and toss anything with more than 3 g per serving. Clear out sauces that have more carbs than you want to spare for a condiment (barbecue, hoisin, and ketchup are likely culprits) and replace them with flavorful low-carb or carb-free products like tamari, liquid aminos, and shoyu. Replace balsamic vinegar (which can have up to 5 g of carbs per tablespoon) with white balsamic (typically 3 g of carbs) or red or white wine vinegar (often 0 g).

Adopt an attitude of self-care.

I counsel a lot of people who are "too busy" to live a healthy lifestyle. They work hard at their jobs, juggle professional demands with family time, and rarely do something just for themselves. Exercise, reading for leisure, and quiet time alone simply don't "fit" in their lives. And preparing a healthy meal? Forget it! Who has time for that?

Well I have news for you: weight loss is about taking care of *you*. It's about reducing your body size and improving your health so that you may add years of well-being to your life! It's about learning to feed yourself well—to *nourish your body*—rather than throw calories of any sort at it to keep it moving to the finish line (nearer every day if you stick to your same routine, ahem!). The sooner you adopt an attitude of self-care, the easier and more successful your diet will become. Make you and your health priority #1 for a change.

Cultivate your inner food snob.

What's one thing in your life that others think you are picky about? Maybe you wouldn't dare buy non-designer shoes or get your hair cut at a chain salon. Take that snobbish attitude and apply it to food. Redefine what you deem is "good enough" for you to eat and make sure that only high-quality, nutritious, low-carb foods fit into that definition. If a food is industrially processed and full of ingredients you can't pronounce, then it likely has tons of calories from sugar and starch as well. The average American gets over half of their calories from processed foods. Most foods built to last on grocery store shelves can do so thanks in part to sweeteners like sugar, high-fructose corn syrup, and the like. Starch improves the volume and texture of certain foods, and is often used as a cheap "filler" so that less of a more expensive item is needed (this practice is common in yogurts and deli meats). You (and your fancy hairdo) are above that.

Use accurate information sources.

Many of the popular nutrition and diet tracking apps and websites use a mix of data sources, some more accurate than others. The most reliable source for nutrient content of whole, unpackaged foods (e.g., chicken breast, broccoli) is the USDA food nutrient database. But because the USDA does not include a wide variety of packaged or restaurant foods, information on such foods in popular diet-tracking apps may be crowd-sourced from app users who want to increase the number of foods in the database. Some of this information is spot-on, and some is dead wrong. A second problem is that different brands of foods have different nutrient compositions, and this variation is not always accounted for in apps. In order to be sure of the carb content of the foods you are eating, it's best to check the labels on the actual foods, as well as restaurant- or brand-produced nutrition information pamphlets.

Find suitable keto substitutes for foods that fit the shape of your day.

For example, say you eat a sandwich every afternoon for lunch so that you can run errands while you eat. Don't try to replace your very convenient and portable sandwich with a delicious chicken breast sautéed in butter and rosemary with a side of broccoli and hollandaise sauce, unless you're *also* willing to take the time to slow down and eat it with a fork and knife. Perhaps that degree of slowing down would be a welcome change in your life.

If that's you, then go for it! If that's too much change for you then you'll have to find other lunch options that fit in your lifestyle. Depending on what you get on your sandwich, you may be able to eat just the inside and leave the bread aside. There are dozens of other suggestions in Chapter 8 "Meal Options."

Read food labels and count your carbs!

If this wasn't clear throughout the book, YOU MUST READ FOOD LABELS. Do not eat anything out of a box or a package unless you know the net carb content for the amount you're eating. Total carbs - fiber = net carbs. Know the number before you take a bite.

Give yourself treats that matter to you.

I discovered this tip one day while I was grating some cheese over my scrambled eggs. I dropped some on the edge of the skillet and it burned. It smelled *sooo* good! I remembered that smell from childhood. It brought me back to the days of making grilled cheese sandwiches, and how the edges where the cheese had burned on the side of the pan were my favorite part. I'd forgotten about that for most of my adulthood. I mean, burnt cheese is rather indulgent... but as I've developed the discipline to forego bread, ice cream, and chocolate, I'd say I'm allowed a bit of a burnt-cheese indulgence every once in a while. So instead of scraping it off the sides of the pan into the trash, now I just throw it on top of whatever I'm eating—*yum*. I encourage you to find something on the keto eating plan that makes you feel blissfully carefree and childlike, and every once in a while give yourself that nice treat.

Look for new recipes and keto-friendly ways to prepare meals.

There are literally thousands of recipes out there for the low carb/ketogenic dieter. Savory meals are easy to prepare in keto-friendly ways, but you may find that you need some inspiration for snacks and desserts. Never fear: there is a world of keto dessert recipes on the web. Many people bake with almond or coconut flour in place of wheat flour and use sugar alcohols and stevia as sweeteners. Check out the resource section of this book (page 290) for URLs to sites with recipes galore. Do you have a chef friend or a friend who loves to cook? Invite him or her to have a day of exploration with you in the kitchen. Stock up on keto-friendly foods and make up your own carb-free specialties! Try some techniques for sauce-making and soup-making. Pull together some fresh ingredients for new takes on salad. Make sure to give dessert a whirl. When you've mastered some favorites, post them on a keto web forum for others to enjoy, too!

Make nutrition and healthy living a new hobby.

Do you read a newspaper or magazine? Start to take an interest in the headlines about diet and health. Once you set out to find these types of stories, chances are you'll see them all the time. Helpful articles like "How to Kick That Sugar Addiction" or "10 Tips for Sticking to That New Diet" should stand out. You may even decide to subscribe to a healthy living magazine, or sign up for a class on low-carb or paleo cooking. See if there's a local low-carb living group in your area, or even a hiking or biking club. Immerse yourself in healthy activities surrounded by healthy people, and you'll keep the weight off.

Find other things to do with your time besides planning your next meal.

A lot of my clients who struggle with overeating are simply too focused on food. These people have some of the same challenges as the "overly busy" people, with one notable trait: every free moment is devoted to thinking about their next snack or meal. They lack fun in their day-to-day responsibilities and consider food a "treat" they offer themselves for having made it through an hour or two of daily boredom. To put it bluntly: this is not an ideal context for weight loss.

Are your thoughts consumed with food? If so, it's best to decide right now to change that. Do you have a hobby? If so, shift some of your snacking time to pursuing it. If not, find one! What else do you like to do besides eat? When your mind is engaged in something you're interested in— knitting, let's say, or gardening, painting, doing crossword puzzles, or fixing gadgets—you will find that thoughts of food come less often and it's easier for you to wait until mealtimes to eat.

CHAPTER 11

Many Uses for the Ketogenic Diet

A ketogenic diet is any diet that causes and maintains ketosis. There are a few different kinds of ketogenic diets in use today, ranging from highly restrictive to more lenient. Some are used by generally healthy individuals for weight loss or to improve body composition, while others are used in clinics or hospital settings as treatment for diseases ranging from severe obesity to cancer to epilepsy and Parkinson's disease. There is a good deal of misinformation out there about the ketogenic diet and ketosis. So while this book describes how to do a moderately restrictive ketogenic diet for weight loss, it may also be helpful to know a bit about various other uses and styles of the diet.

"Atkins" Is a Household Name

Dr. Robert Atkins is arguably the father of the modern ketogenic diet for weight loss. But is the ketogenic diet the same as the Atkins diet? Yes and no. The Atkins diet takes advantage of ketosis to burn fat and speed weight loss, so the approach to metabolic manipulation is the same. What distinguishes the Atkins diet is mainly the structure of the plan and how the diet is perceived by the public.

Atkins is a specific program that has four phases and a maintenance phase, starting with a ketogenic phase called Induction. Each phase has allowed and disallowed foods. Phase 1 restricts carbs to 20 g per day *at most*; Phase 2 allows 30–80 g (the lower end of this range will keep many dieters in ketosis); Phase 3 recommends increasing carb intake by 10 g at a time as long as weight loss or maintenance (whichever the dieter wants) persists; and Phase 4 focuses on maintaining weight by adjusting carb intake as needed. Thus, Atkins guides dieters first through a ketogenic diet for rapid weight loss and then progresses to a less restrictive eating pattern that is considered low-carb compared to the average diet, but which is no longer ketogenic above a certain threshold (about 50–60 g of carbs per day).

It was probably a combination of Atkins diet marketing that highlights "indulgent" foods (like steak and butter) allowed on the diet, as well as the severe restriction of carbs in Phase 1, that created the public perception of the Atkins diet as one in which you eat large amounts of saturated fat and very few (if any) vegetables. This is hardly the picture of a healthful diet, and it was never intended to be a long-term eating strategy—even on Atkins.

Benefits of a High-Fat Diet

Interview with Valerie Berkowitz, MS, RD, CDE, CDN

The Atkins diet ultimately helped millions of people lose weight and gain other health benefits. I spoke with registered dietitian Valerie Berkowitz, who worked with Dr. Atkins at his health clinic in New York City and who continues to use very-low-carbohydrate and ketogenic diets in her current practice.

How did you first come to work with the ketogenic diet in your nutrition practice?

I worked with Dr. Atkins in his practice and then branched out on my own after his death. I witnessed firsthand the benefits patients experienced using a high-fat diet. I have been using this diet for over twenty years on my patients, my family, and myself. The research is only now catching up and I am happy I did not wait for it because I have helped change people's lives for the better through all these years!

What, if anything, surprised you about the diet or its effects?

I was surprised with it all. I was a vegetarian, and conventionally trained by the same RDs who insist this is the most unhealthy diet around. I thought people would be very, very sick—but they were not! Health parameters and mood improved, motivation was high due to the rapid weight loss...it seemed like a miracle and for many people it was. Three main things stood out:

1. There were no complaints of cravings, hunger, or issues with appetite...patients were reporting they were forgetting to eat lunch.

2. It seemed to be a corrective diet, correcting metabolic abnormalities (metabolic syndrome, diabetes, polycystic ovary syndrome [PCOS], heart disease, high blood pressure, cholesterol) and various additional issues like skin, sleep, headache, focus and brain fog, GI issues, attention deficit disorder (ADD).

3. I was surprised at just how healthy and nutrient-dense a low-carb, high-fat diet was. I was unable to recommend low-fat snack packs, yogurt, pretzels, baked chips just because they were low in fat because after reading the labels (even in infant zwieback crackers) I believed that the trans fat and fructose in these products were worse for health than the natural fat in an avocado, shredded coconut, or olives.

When do you recommend a ketogenic diet to your clients?

I work with my clients based on their preference, not mine. I explain how both low-fat and high-fat plans work (burning fat or glucose) and let them choose. Most choose a ketogenic diet when they understand the facts. I ask the skeptics to do it for a week. If I'm wrong and they do not feel better and lose weight, we try something else. Nine-and-a-half times out of ten they ask to stay on the strictest phase of my diet, the Stubborn Fat Fix, for a longer time.

Many dietitians recommend a low-fat diet for weight loss and assert that eating too much fat will give you heart disease. Do you agree?

Yes, they are right. But only when they are talking about high amounts of fat in the presence of high amounts of carbs. When carbs are reduced so the body burns fat as a primary fuel source (similar to an athlete/marathon runner or body builder) this is absolutely false. This is why the debate is ridiculous; they are not comparing apples to apples and refuse to understand or admit that this difference is critical in how the body manages nutrients.

Quite frankly it does not really matter if I agree. This claim, like all the claims against ketogenic diets, is 100 percent unfounded. The research that many claim supports the myth that very-low-carbohydrate diets lead to heart disease are the studies that do not use a fat-based metabolism or ketosis (meaning, they don't go low enough in carbs or use the diet for long enough to maintain ketosis).

The research shows that sugar (100 percent of carbs convert to sugar in the blood) and low-fat diets can lead to heart disease (Darlene Dreon has done good research on this point). So it seems prudent that at least both diets deserve a fair shot.

Another point is that if you are promoting health and well-being you want to nourish the body with fat and the absorption of fat-soluble vitamins to support normal body functions (i.e., sex hormones, nerves, brain, body cells), prevent advanced glycation end products (AGEs), and maintain a steady state of insulin and glucose, among many other things—not just focus on heart disease and ignore all the other health problems that can accompany low-fat diets.

Does a ketogenic diet really help people lose more weight and keep it off? A lot of studies say that the weight comes back after a year. What's your experience?

Just like with any diet, if you go back to poor old dietary habits, you gain it back. For those who make it a lifestyle (myself included), the results last, and sticking to the plan is not so hard when you feel good; that is the motivation to stick with it.

Valerie Berkowitz is Nutrition Director at the Center for Balanced Health (www.centerforbalancedhealth.com) in New York City and the author of The Stubborn Fat Fix: Eat Right to Lose Weight and Cure Metabolic Burnout without Hunger or Exercise *(Rodale, 2009). She was previously Supervisor of Education and Research at the Atkins Center for Complementary Medicine and Atkins Heath and Medical Information Services.*

Side-Stepping Brain Malfunction by Eliminating Glucose

The widest application of ketogenic diets in the last twenty years has been for pediatric epilepsy. In many cases, after a year or two on the diet, children are cured of their seizure disorders completely. The ketogenic diet seems to work just as well for adults with epileptic disorders, although it is less often used with that population because it is believed to be too difficult for adults to follow. Unlike the ketogenic diet for weight loss, this version of the diet requires food portions to be measured and weighed, and nutrients to be calculated precisely. It requires strict adherence, and is almost always done under medical supervision.

A tremendous amount of research has been done to determine exactly how the diet works for seizure control, and it is still something of a mystery. The answer certainly lies in manipulating brain metabolism. Normally, the brain uses glucose for energy. But on a ketogenic diet, when glucose is

scarce, the brain shifts to using ketones. It has been demon-
strated in animal studies that ketones can mend neurons,
and they have an anti-inflammatory effect on the brain.
Another theory suggests that ketones bypass some of the
damaged pathways used in brain metabolism of glucose.
Whatever the mechanism, this change appears to benefit
a number of neurological conditions, including Alzheimer's,
Parkinson's, and even damage from traumatic brain Injury.

The potential of the ketogenic diet to prevent, treat, and
even cure a wide range of brain-related diseases cannot be
overstated. A thorough discussion of the subject is well
beyond the scope of this book, but if you'd like to learn
more, visit the website of the Charlie Foundation, an organization devoted to raising awareness about the ketogenic
diet for neurological disorders, at www.charliefoundation
.org. The site also provides helpful resources to the average
ketogenic dieter, including ketogenic recipes, a list of carb-
free medications, and more. (See page 293 for more information about resources provided by the Charlie Foundation.)

Cancer Cells Can't Use Ketones

You may have heard that "cancer thrives on glucose."
Cancer cells use glucose for energy. Rapidly growing tumor
cells typically use glucose *200 times faster* than normal cells.
There is some evidence that "starving" cancer cells with a
low-carbohydrate diet can slow the growth of tumor cells.
Also, insulin promotes tumor cell growth, thus a low-
carbohydrate diet may further inhibit tumor growth in part
by reducing insulin levels.

Cancer as a Metabolic Disease

Interview with Thomas N. Seyfried

I spoke with Dr. Thomas N. Seyfried, PhD, Professor of Biology at Boston College and author of the textbook *Cancer as a Metabolic Disease: On the Origin, Management, and Prevention of Cancer* (Wiley, 2012). Dr. Seyfried has been researching and teaching in the field of neurogenetics, neurochemistry, and cancer for over 25 years and has published over 150 scientific articles.

Please describe your work / mission.

My research focuses on gene environmental interactions related to complex diseases, such as epilepsy, autism, brain cancer, and neurodegenerative diseases.

Your work rests on the theory that cancer is a metabolic disorder. How is that different from other theories?

The general theory today is that cancer is a disease of the DNA in the cell nucleus. Under this theory, cancer is thought to arise from mutations in the DNA leading to uncontrolled cell growth.

The metabolic theory states that cancer arises from damage to cellular respiration (mitochondria). This leads to a shift in cellular energy metabolism from respiration to fermentation. Fermentation is a primitive form of energy metabolism that existed before the appearance of oxygen on the planet. Under this theory, the DNA mutations are considered downstream effects of abnormal energy metabolism.

The strongest evidence against the nuclear gene theory and supporting the metabolic theory of cancer comes from the nuclear transfer experiments. Tumors do not form when the nucleus of the tumor cell, containing mutations, is placed in normal cell cytoplasm containing normal mitochondria. On the other hand, tumors can form when a normal nucleus is placed into the cytoplasm from a tumor cell. These findings indicate that nuclear gene mutations are not the drivers of cancer, and that normal mitochondria in the cytoplasm can suppress tumor formation.

What makes a ketogenic diet effective for treatment of cancer?

All tumor cells depend to some degree on fermentation energy for growth and survival. Normal cells depend on respiration for energy. The dependency (of cancer cells) on fermentation for energy comes from defects in the cellular mitochondria, which are responsible for respiration. The major fuel for fermentation is glucose. The low-carbohydrate, high-fat ketogenic diet will lower availability of glucose and will elevate ketones in the body. The ketones are produced from metabolism of fats. Healthy mitochondria are needed to metabolize ketone bodies for energy. Mitochondria are unhealthy in the majority of cancer cells. Consequently, the ketogenic diet will lower the major carbohydrate fuel (glucose) for cancer cell fermentation while elevating ketones, which the tumor cells cannot use for energy. This is a simple way, in principle, of starving the tumor cells while enhancing the health of normal body cells.

Is there any chance that following a ketogenic or very-low-carb diet can prevent cancer?

Cancer arises from damage to the mitochondria. Any diet that enhances the health and vitality of mitochondria will prevent cancer. Water-only therapeutic fasting for several days will also enhance the health of mitochondria.

Where do you recommend people find out more?

We have published several articles in open-access journals like *Nutrition & Metabolism* and *PLOS ONE*. The general public can easily access these articles free from the web. My book, *Cancer as a Metabolic Disease*, is also available through Amazon and Barnes & Noble.

What else do you think is important to know about the ketogenic diet and cancer?

It is important to recognize that the ketogenic diet should not be considered a "cure" for cancer. The KD, when administered in restricted amounts and under appropriate supervision, can slow tumor growth without toxicity to the patient. The KD might even be more effective in managing cancer when combined with non-toxic drugs or even with low doses of toxic chemotherapy. The KD should be viewed as a medical therapy.

Every cancer patient should be made aware of the non-toxic options for cancer management. Standard treatments can effectively manage some cancers, but cannot manage all cancers. According to the American Cancer Society, over 1,500 people die each day from cancer. Cancers that spread or metastasize remain largely unmanageable using standard treatments. Cancer patients should know their options and choose for themselves the treatment that is best.

The Ketone-Fueled Super Soldier

The military has been looking into the ketogenic diet as a way to enhance the ability of naval divers to carry out missions deep under sea. These divers have a high risk of seizures because of their specialized breathing equipment, which, unlike typical diving equipment, circulates gases in such a way as to make the equipment silent; but this exposes the soldiers to levels of oxygen that are toxic and often results in seizures.

Applying the Ketogenic Diet to Real-Life Problems
Interview with Dominic D'Agostino

I spoke with Dominic D'Agostino, PhD, Assistant Professor at the University of South Florida and Morsani College of Medicine, who researches applications of the ketogenic diet to this and other exciting purposes—like sending people to Mars!

Please describe your work with the ketogenic diet.

Most of my research has been prompted by needs from the military. They're interested in preventing seizures in divers who get "oxygen toxicity" when diving. My mission was to predict why this occurred and prevent it. I started looking into different anti-seizure strategies, and I stumbled across the ketogenic diet. I didn't know the history of the diet. Fasting has been reported to control seizures even back to the time of Hippocrates in 400 BC. The ketogenic diet mimics fasting, and there's something about being in a fasted state that shifts brain metabolism. Ketones provide a source of energy for the brain, and they protect cells from damage by oxidative stress. It reduces the effects of stress in other tissues, too, not just the brain, and makes them more metabolically resilient in situations of high energy demands or environmental stress. The military is interested in using this strategy to make a super soldier—one who can withstand high altitude and deep sea diving without ill effects.

One of the more interesting applications is the use of ketones for astronaut safety and resilience. For example, we want to get astronauts to Mars. But Mars is far away—it's about 1,000 times farther than the moon. It will take two years or more to get there. During this time astronauts get hit with a lot of radiation, and that's dangerous. So NASA is looking for ways to protect them. You can think about building a bigger shield around the ship, but it's a lot of weight, and it's very expensive. So now they are looking at physiological/biochemical ways to preserve cell health under radiation. Ketones protect body tissues and the brain from radiation. They also help you think better under conditions of environmental stress, for example, where pressure and oxygen levels are lower. The government has done some research that shows that animal cells exposed to ketones will live longer than normal cells when they are also exposed to radiation. I was really excited when NASA called me to talk about this! These are some of the things that I never thought would evolve from our ketone research, but they are happening.

What do you think of the ketogenic diet for the average person?

There's a really potent mechanism behind this diet. It's not for everyone, but some form of carbohydrate restriction is beneficial for most people, especially people who are struggling with long-term poor blood sugar control. I think it's important that people are aware that the diet is pretty flexible. When you have fat to work with you have a lot of ability to create flavor. There are even ways to make ketogenic ice cream, cookies, and muffins. One of my favorite ketogenic desserts is a Chocolate Coconut Custard Ice Cream (page 286) I make myself.

What's your definition of a ketogenic diet?

I started hearing about the "ketogenic" diet in 2008 in the fitness community, but it was really just a low-carb, high-protein diet used in the fitness community that wasn't actually ketogenic.

My definition of a ketogenic diet is an elevation of blood ketone levels. In order to achieve that you need to restrict your carbs, moderate your protein levels, and give your body fat. Everyone's going to have a different carb threshold. If you're active and younger, you'll have a higher tolerance. Carb tolerance reduces as we age. I think the dietary guidelines should reflect that and recommend a trend toward lower-carb diets as we age. Of course, I'm an advocate for very-low-carb diets in general.

Maybe it sounds obsessive but I'm an advocate of self-experimentation. I think it's most helpful for someone to monitor their blood glucose response to meals to help them learn their carb tolerance. It's the blood glucose and insulin rise and fall that triggers hunger, and I see how it can become a vicious cycle for people trying to lose weight. People will have more control if they take it upon themselves to learn how foods affect their blood glucose. A blood glucose monitor is available at any pharmacy. It may seem extreme, but diabetics do it. It's just taking blood a few times a day. There are really easy ways to do it nowadays. It's a technology available to everyone. I know people who were obese and got started measuring their glucose levels after eating, and they were able to get their weight under control by monitoring and then adding carbs back into their diet—even up to 100 g a day. They were able to include things they like a lot, such as chocolate and blueberries. What happened was these people gained tight control over their metabolic physiology and had more freedom in eating and staying lean.

How do your family and friends react to your diet?

My parents live in New Jersey and I grew up in an Italian family eating pasta. When I first started my mom was confused and just thought it was a weird thing that Dominic was doing. She called and said, "When you come home, what are you going to eat?" And she would ask, "Are you eating normal now?"

Generally, people just think it's really interesting, and it's a source of conversation. It doesn't socially isolate me. I have friends that have epilepsy that need to follow it strictly, and they will actually bring a scale to the restaurant and do some quick calculations to determine the macronutrient profile. Restaurants are usually very accommodating.

Many friends have gone in this direction now and have derived a lot of benefit from it. They have started advocating it, and people are calling me and asking about it. My family has actually started to embrace it. They are replacing a lot of the bread with vegetables, and they have started pushing out a lot of the starches and definitely the sugars. Now my friends and family are pretty excited about it. They ask me what sort of research studies are in the pipeline.

Do you ever eat pasta? If so, what happens?

Sometimes, if I'm traveling in Europe or Italy, I'll eat a forkful. I really have an appreciation of foods from other cultures, so I like to try things and be respectful when I'm there. Sometimes, if you arrive in a new place, people will have prepared a whole meal for you! I have carb loaded before in situations like these. But I tolerate carbs well.

Dominic D'Agostino's fascinating Ted Talk on the metabolic benefits of ketones, titled "Starving Cancer," can be viewed on YouTube.com. His website, ketonutrition.org, is an excellent resource where you can learn more about ketogenic nutrition, find online sources for keto-friendly foods and ketone supplements, and access videos, podcasts, and articles from ketogenic diet experts.

CHAPTER 12

Keto-Paleo Crossover and the Popularity of Low-Carb Eating

It's no secret that to maintain weight loss you must integrate the behaviors that helped you lose weight into a feasible long-term lifestyle. It's especially helpful if that lifestyle is practiced by others around you, both family and friends and those closest to you, as well as society at large.

The Paleo Diet: A Ketogenic Dieter's New Best Friend

Today, in 2015, the ketogenic dieter is in good company with the paleo diet. The paleo or "ancestral" diet is, without question, the lowest-carb, highest-fat diet super-trend we've seen in decades. The major difference between a ketogenic diet and a paleo diet is that a paleo diet focuses on types of foods rather than nutrients, while a ketogenic diet is based on upping fat and cutting carbs, regardless of the foods eaten. A paleo diet isn't necessarily ketogenic (some people practice it that way, but most do not), and a ketogenic diet doesn't *technically* restrict food groups.

If, for example, you wanted to consume two teaspoons of table sugar (9 g of carbs) each day while still staying within your carb allotment, that would technically still be ketogenic. A paleo dieter won't touch table sugar, period, but may be comfortable eating many more than 9 g of sugar in the form of dates or honey. In practice, though, the food groups that paleo cuts out happen to be the same ones that the ketogenic diet cuts out, with a couple of exceptions. As you move from your highly carb-restricted diet to perhaps a more lenient approach, you may find that you have no trouble maintaining your weight somewhat above your ketogenic threshold. If this is you, you may likely end up eating a diet that can be labeled as "paleo." So if you're concerned about making the leap to eating slightly more carbs—say 75–150 g per day—on your own, and you're looking to latch on to another structured diet plan to help you through the transition, then paleo is your ticket.

A paleo diet centers on the whole, unprocessed foods that were available to humans before the advent of agriculture (and *well before* industrial food manufacturing) 12,000 years ago. (This is why paleo is also sometimes called *ancestral* or *primal*, in reference to the diet of our ancestors). In explicit terms, paleo embraces meat, fish, fowl, vegetables, fruits, and nuts, while grains, legumes, and dairy are out. The paleo diet says "no, thank you" to most processed foods, although things like tomato sauce and olive oil, which undergo some minimal processing, are permitted.

A key difference between the paleo and ketogenic diets is that paleo allows starchy vegetables and fruit, and does not allow dairy. Despite this distinction, the two diets are still close cousins. Some paleo practitioners do consider dairy an acceptable food in small amounts, a principle that the ketogenic diet shares. And although paleo *permits* starches and sugars from whole food sources, the philosophy of the diet is one of moderation, not excess. A paleo diet says "sure, sweet potatoes and apples are okay to eat, but pace yourself, because they have a lot of sugar."

"Paleo-friendly" food products and menus are popping up everywhere, and this is one reason why jumping on board the paleo train is a smart strategy for maintaining the weight loss you achieved on the ketogenic diet. If you've come across the Net Carb Zero bread in your grocery store you probably noticed that the company that makes this product also makes a number of products labeled "paleo"; in fact, a good majority of the new, very-low-carb food products out there are being manufactured specifically to meet the market demands of the paleo dieting community—of which there are (just a guess) likely thousands of new members each day.

It's hard to look at a magazine or website about diet and nutrition nowadays and *not* notice the uber popularity of the paleo trend. If I were writing this book ten years ago, I wouldn't even be bringing it up; back then, "Paleolithic nutrition" was a term used only in professional literature by anthropologists, evolutionary biologists, and the like. But today, paleo is the topic on everyone's tongue, and, luckily for the low-carb dieter, the movement seems only to be gaining steam.

Advice from a Low-Carb Eater

Interview with Mark Sisson

I spoke with Mark Sisson, author of *The Primal Blue print* and creator of *Marks Daily Apple: Primal Living in the Modern World*, a mega-popular website focused on promoting the paleo diet and lifestyle. Mark's site provides thoughtful commentary on the role of fat, sugar, and starch in human health, among other things. Find him at www.MarksDailyApple.com.

What's your philosophy on health?

Health is the most important asset that we all have, and we have far more control over it than most people imagine. It comes down to the choices we make.

What are your thoughts on fat in the diet?

Humans have a "factory setting" that allows us to be very efficient at burning fat. We have lost that skill because of the preponderance of sugar and carbs all around. The human body doesn't want to waste energy, so because you've spent your whole life providing your brain with glucose in the form of pancakes, orange juice, etc., it down-regulates all the enzymes and pathways that are involved in fat metabolism, and makes you a sugar-burner.

The goal is to reaccess that setting that allows us to become a fat-burning machine. You have to understand that fat is not bad. To vilify fat is a big mistake in terms of crafting a healthy lifestyle for yourself. I believe that the less glucose you burn over a lifetime, the better. There's an amount of carbohydrate that's appropriate for everyone, and to exceed that is to flirt with metabolic dysfunction—whether that's a little bit of weight gain or full-blown diabetes.

If you get rid of all the processed foods and the sugars and reduce the grains, cut out pasta, cereal, cookies, crackers, and chips, you're left with choices that include copious amounts of vegetables, some fruits, and the occasional starchy tuber. You would be hard pressed to exceed 150–200 g of carbs on a diet like this.

Do you recommend a ketogenic diet?

I think ketogenic diets are a good thing for a short time for most people, and some people have to stick with them for a long time. I do what I do and talk about food because I love food and I love living, and I don't want to deprive myself of any food. I'm a fan of cyclic ketogenic diets, where you ease into and out of a ketogenic state. You spend some time eating 50–100 g per day, which sends signals to the body that you're going to go keto-genic, and then in the transition out you reintroduce foods with some more carbs. Don't go from ketogenic to eating 450 g of carbs per day. The idea is to achieve an enhanced level of fat-burning and maintain that ability.

What sort of diet do you follow?

I am a low-carb eater compared to the rest of the world. I'm in the 150–200 g range for carbohydrate intake. But I don't want to withhold any foods if I don't have to, and because I maintain good body composition for a man my age, I don't feel the need to go deep into ketosis. I feel as though I've created the metabolic machinery to go a day-and-a-half without eating, if for whatever reason I need to do that. But I won't forego the vegetables or the bowl of fruit because it will take me out of ketosis. But if I had metabolic issues (such as excess weight or insulin resistance), I would be accessing this technology all the time!

A Food Environment Fit for a Low-Carb Dieter

Nutrition educators understand that an individual is not solely responsible for his or her food choices, using his or her taste buds as the singular guiding force toward the odd Big Mac or Twix bar floating in a sea of kale and cucumbers. We know that there are other forces of influence besides what are known as "taste preferences," and that access to healthful foods is usually the primary factor determining whether a person, in any given instance, will ultimately eat healthful foods. When we're asked what the secret is to persuading people to eat healthier diets, some of us in the nutrition field like to say: "Make the healthy choice the easy choice."

The phrase "food environment" accounts for what's available to eat in places where we usually do so, as well as which foods are encouraged by advertising, peer groups, and general visibility. This includes seemingly trivial things like which foods in the grocery store are shelved at eye level and which we have to reach for. These factors play a huge role in shaping an individual's food choices. Improving the food environment by making more nutritious foods available in our grocery stores, restaurants, cafeterias, vending machines, schools, and so on, can help make "the healthy choice" a whole lot easier.

The same holds true if you're trying to follow a specific type of diet: the easier it is to find the foods permitted on your plan, the more successful you will be in sticking to it. Luckily for the low-carb dieter, the current wave of nutritional advice is geared toward higher-fat, lower-carb eating patterns, and carb-free or very low-carb foods are available almost everywhere. Today's food environment is quickly becoming an optimal one for the ketogenic dieter.

CHAPTER 13

Recipes

This chapter consists of a handful of recipes that I found myself using regularly on the ketogenic diet and think will be quite useful for anyone starting out. For the most part, they are simple preparations of keto staples (like guacamole) and keto adaptations of commonly eaten dishes (like mashed potatoes); and, of course there are some suggestions for keto desserts. I either created the recipes myself, tweaked them from old standards, or gathered them from friends and colleagues familiar with low-carb cooking.

This chapter will get you started, and as you spend more time on the diet you may want to expand your keto cooking repertoire. Paleo cookbooks are an invaluable resource, and you will easily find keto-acceptable entrées and non-starchy vegetable recipes in most any cookbook as long as the dishes do not contain flours or grains. (Any meat-based entree is usually fair game—no pun intended!). You can also check out the recipe resources at the end of this chapter. And don't forget to ask kitchen-savvy friends for new ideas!

CAULIFLOWER MASHED POTATOES

Cauliflower is a magic vegetable. Before the diet, I'd never given it any thought. Although I knew it had super cancer-fighting nutrients, it just seemed…boring. Being on the ketogenic diet forced me to look for new sides to make with dinner, so one day I decided to give this a try.

I'd gotten the recipe for this silky, creamy dish from Devon Dionne of Open Sky Fitness in Los Angeles. Devon is a former professional dancer, a Certified Holistic Health Coach, and a GYROTONIC instructor.

1 head cauliflower

1 tablespoon olive oil

2 tablespoons chopped fresh rosemary

1 tablespoon butter

2 tablespoons heavy cream

2 tablespoons unsweetened almond milk

1 teaspoon sea salt, or more as needed

Break the cauliflower into florets and steam or *briefly* boil until soft. Heat olive oil in a skillet and add chopped rosemary, cooking 1–2 minutes; then add butter and melt, and add cauliflower to pan to coat with seasoning. Cook 1 minute more, then mash cauliflower with a potato masher in the pan.

Pour contents of pan into blender, add heavy cream and almond milk while blending. The mixture will be creamy on the bottom and chunkier on top, so it's best to stop the blender and mix with a spoon once or twice. If you make sure to do this and it's still too chunky you can add more cream or almond milk, but if you add too much it will be runny. Add salt while processing, to taste.

Devon says she brings this mash to holiday parties "and guests don't even notice the difference. They only compliment on how light, fluffy, and delicious the 'potatoes' taste." Ha!

● ● ●

ITALIAN SPICY SAUSAGE AND BROCCOLI RABE

This is a one-dish meal based on the Italian leafy green, broccoli rabe. Broccoli rabe is a cross between broccoli and something like kale. It has small broccoli florets sticking off of leafy stems. It comes in a bunch like other leafy greens. A unique feature of broccoli rabe is its exceedingly high fiber-to-total-carb ratio: 90 percent of the carbohydrate in this vegetable is in the form of fiber. An entire bunch of cooked broccoli rabe has just 1.5 g of net carbs! You can substitute kale, mustard greens, or any other hearty green in the dish—but you'll be adding more carbs.

> 1 bunch broccoli rabe
>
> 4 tablespoons olive oil
>
> 1–2 teaspoons red pepper flakes
>
> 1 teaspoon sea salt
>
> 1 pound hot Italian sausage links
>
> grated Parmesan cheese (optional)

Wash the broccoli rabe. Cut off and discard the bottom 2 inches of the stems. Chop the vegetable into roughly 1-inch pieces. Heat olive oil in a large skillet, preferably with high sides. Add the broccoli rabe, salt, and red pepper flakes and sauté for 4–5 minutes or until the greens have softened and the leafy parts are wilted. Remove the broccoli rabe and set aside.

Add sausages to the skillet, browning on each side until cooked through, about 10 minutes. Check for doneness by cutting into the sausage; cook a few minutes more if needed. The sausages may break apart and crumble while cooking, and that's okay. Once they have cooled you can slice them into 1-inch-thick pieces or crumble them and mix into the broccoli rabe. Grate Parmesan cheese on top, if desired.

This is a filling and tasty dish that's a meal on its own, and it's a big crowd-pleaser at potlucks (except among vegetarians).

● ●

SALT-AND-PEPPER CHICKEN

This is the fastest, tastiest chicken recipe I know. You squeeze as many chicken pieces as can fit into the pan, and the fact that they're snuggled together keeps the juices in and prevents them from drying out. Use coarse sea salt and fresh cracked pepper for a crunchy coating.

> 4–6 chicken breasts
>
> 2 tablespoons oil (coconut and olive are good options)
>
> 1 tablespoon coarse sea salt (or more)
>
> 1 tablespoon fresh cracked pepper (or more)

Cut chicken breasts into 3–4-inch pieces. Thin out any pieces that are thicker than the others by cutting horizontally. Your goal is to get the pieces roughly the same thickness; otherwise, some will cook much faster than others.

Heat the oil in a large, heavy skillet (cast iron is ideal). Place the chicken pieces in the pan so that they cover the cooking surface and touch the sides of the pan, leaving no room in between them.

Sprinkle the salt from high above the pan so that it distributes evenly, then crack a good deal of pepper over the chicken pieces. Let the pieces cook on this side until the bottom begins to brown. Turn pieces over and repeat sprinkling with salt and pepper. Don't be timid with the seasoning!

Serve the chicken on its own with side vegetables, or cover with any sauce you like. It goes well with garlic or herb mayonnaise. Use leftover pieces the next day in a salad or with vegetables for lunch.

> Tip: To check for doneness, cut into a thick part of the breast. The color should be white, with no pink. If some pieces are less thick than others, it's a good idea to remove those first so that they do not get overdone.

● ● ●

ALBONDIGAS DE ESPINACA (MEATBALLS WITH SPINACH)

I'm not a huge meat eater, and one of my biggest challenges was swapping out the rice and beans that are part of my Spanish–Middle Eastern heritage for carbohydrate-free, animal-based proteins.

So as not to give up fully on my cultural food preferences, I dug up some old recipes from my childhood. Here's my grandma's recipe for spinach meatballs, or Albondigas de Espinaca, with almond meal in place of the breadcrumbs.

1 ½ cups fresh spinach leaves

1 pound ground lamb, veal, or beef, or a mix of these

3 tablespoons almond meal (or ground almond flour)

2 eggs

¾ teaspoon salt

¼ teaspoon ground nutmeg

pepper

4 tablespoons olive or grapeseed oil, for frying

Wilt the spinach leaves in a pan on low heat, about 2 minutes. When it's cool, drain and squeeze out the remaining water.

Put all the ingredients, except the cooking oil, in a food processor and blend to a paste. Shape into little meatballs and fry in the oil until brown on all sides.

● ●

KITCHEN SINK SALAD

There is really nothing easier than tossing a bunch of ingredients onto a big bed of lettuce and adding a dressing on top.

pre-washed greens

tomatoes

cucumbers

basil or mint

olives

hard cheese (for grating)

protein component

sesame seeds (optional)

Throw half a bag of pre-washed greens, such as baby spinach or arugula, in a big bowl and slice in some tomatoes, cucumbers, and basil or mint. Add olives, slicing them into pieces. Grate a hard cheese like Parmesan or sharp cheese into the mix to make the salad more flavorful. Add a protein item, such as chicken, salmon, or tofu (maybe you have some left over from the night before), or some omega-3-rich canned Portuguese sardines or mackerel.

If someone is joining you and you want the salad to look pretty, sprinkle some sesame seeds on top. Use the simplest vinaigrette (see recipe on page 184) to dress the salad.

● ●

BROCCOLI IN COCONUT OIL

Most people steam or roast broccoli to get it soft enough to their liking. I prefer to sauté, just because it's faster than roasting and tastier than steaming. I do not know why the combination of broccoli with coconut oil is so delicious, but I urge you to try it and decide for yourself.

1 head broccoli

2 tablespoons coconut oil for cooking, plus 1 tablespoon for finishing the plate

2–3 tablespoons water

sea salt, to taste

Cut the broccoli florets small, so they are about 2 inches long and about 1 inch wide (don't worry if there are some smaller pieces as well). Heat 2 tablespoons of coconut oil in a pan on high heat and add the broccoli florets. They should sizzle. Coat them well with the oil and cook until they start to brown on one side. Cook for 2 more minutes, making sure to turn the less browned sides of the florets toward the surface of the pan. Add 2 tablespoons of water and *cover the pan* to trap the steam. This will soften the broccoli. Cook 2 to 3 minutes more. If broccoli is still too firm or if it starts to burn, add a bit more water and cover again. When the broccoli is almost done, remove the lid to evaporate the water completely. Place the warm broccoli in a bowl and top with the last tablespoon of coconut oil and sea salt, to taste. Mix well.

● ●

EASY GUACAMOLE

Guacamole is simple to make and great keto food to have on hand, as avocado is mainly fat. You don't even need a recipe; just smash a ripe avocado with some sea salt and lime, and a touch of cayenne if you'd like some heat.

You can always add chopped jalapeño, cilantro, onion, tomato, and/or garlic if you're in the mood. Mix and let sit for an hour in the fridge. If it's bland, add more salt and/or lime juice. It's impossible to go wrong making guacamole. If the flavor isn't outstanding, next time use a riper avocado.

● ●

SPICED NUTS

It's always a good idea to keep these around for a much more exciting snack then just a handful of nuts alone.

coconut oil or melted butter, to coat

1–2 cups of walnuts, pecans, and/or almonds

salt, to taste

dry herb or spices of your choice, to taste

Put 3–4 tablespoons of coconut oil or butter in a bowl. Coconut oil will liquefy almost immediately at room temperature; if using butter, microwave on high for 8–10 seconds, or melt in a saucepan over low heat for just a bit longer than that (watch the butter closely and remove from heat when it's nearly liquefied). Add 1–2 cups of walnuts, pecans, almonds, or all three, and coat with the oil. Add a good dose of salt and mix well. Add a dry herb, like rosemary or Herbs de Provence, or something smoky, like smoked paprika and a touch of cayenne, or some cinnamon and a touch of cacao—you get the idea! Mix well. Roast in the oven on low heat for about 15 minutes, checking often to avoid burning.

Sauces & Dressings

● ●

TURMERIC VINAIGRETTE FOR SALADS

Turmeric is prized in Indian traditions for its extraordinary medicinal properties. Studies demonstrate that turmeric reduces inflammation, helps fight infection, and even slows the growth of cancer cells. Systemic inflammation is both a cause and an effect of weight gain, and reducing inflammation can aid weight loss and improve overall health. This dressing makes it easy to get turmeric into your daily diet.

> ½ cup white balsamic vinegar
>
> 1 tablespoon Dijon mustard
>
> 1 teaspoon turmeric
>
> 1 teaspoon sea salt
>
> 1 cup olive oil

Mix vinegar, mustard, turmeric, and salt in a blender for a few seconds, then add oil and blend a few second more until mixed. Store in a jar in the refrigerator for up to three weeks.

Use as a salad dressing. To use as a sauce for meat or vegetables, reduce the vinegar by half.

● ●

BASIL PESTO FOR ANYTHING

Fresh pesto makes anything delicious. I like to use pesto on top of chicken or tofu, in an omelet, or on kelp noodles. (For kelp noodles, dilute pesto by stirring in 1 to 2 tablespoons of cooking water, then tossing noodles into the sauce.)

2 cups fresh basil leaves (no stems)

½ cup olive oil

3 tablespoons pine nuts or walnuts

2 garlic cloves

salt and pepper, to taste

½ cup grated Parmesan cheese

Place basil leaves in a food processor or blender. Add the oil, nuts, garlic, salt, and pepper and blend to a fine texture. Add Parmesan and blend for a few seconds more.

● ●

LEMON-TURMERIC CREAM SAUCE FOR CHICKEN OR FISH

One of the fastest ways to add fat and flavor to cooked food is to make a sauce in the pan as soon as you're done cooking your protein item. This recipe works perfectly for sautéed chicken or fish.

protein item, such as chicken or fish

¾ cup heavy cream

juice of 1 lemon

1 teaspoon turmeric

sea salt and fresh cracked pepper

As soon as you're done sautéing your protein item, remove that from the pan and place in a deep dish (for collecting juices). Add the cream, lemon, and turmeric to the original pan and bring to a boil. Add in any juices that have collected under the protein. Simmer until thickened to your liking, stirring often, and adding salt and pepper to taste. Makes enough to cover 4 chicken breasts or fish fillets.

● ● ●

MISO-SESAME DRESSING FOR TOFU AND VEGETABLES

This recipe is adapted from the fantastic cooking blog, Smitten Kitchen. While the site overall is not low-carb territory, this particular sauce makes a great addition to any keto fridge. It requires some Asian ingredients, so it's a good excuse to go to the Asian grocery store and explore the huge variety of carb-free foods there (noodles made of tofu, exotic mushrooms, spicy pickled vegetables). I've left out the 1 tablespoon of honey (17 g of carbs) called for in the original recipe, but you can easily add back ½ teaspoon for a hint of sweetness and still keep under 5 g of carbs per serving. The recipe makes about 1 cup of dressing.

1 tablespoon minced fresh ginger

1 small garlic clove, minced

1 tablespoon white miso

2 tablespoons tahini or other nut butter

¼ cup rice vinegar

2 tablespoons toasted sesame oil

2 tablespoons olive oil

Combine everything in a blender and mix until smooth. If it's too thick for your taste, blend in 2 tablespoons of unsweetened almond milk.

Use on top of baked or sautéed tofu or vegetables.

● ●

CHIMICHURRI SAUCE FOR STEAK

Chimichurri is an Argentinian sauce made of fresh herbs and vinegar. It has a fresh, tart flavor that balances out the rich, buttery taste of steak.

    1 cup chopped fresh parsley

    1 cup chopped fresh cilantro

    ⅔ cup olive oil

    6 tablespoons white vinegar

    2 tablespoons minced garlic

    sea salt and fresh cracked pepper, to taste

    1 teaspoon red pepper flakes, for some heat
    (optional)

Mix all ingredients together in a bowl. If you prefer a finer texture and don't like to chop vegetables, put the parsley, cilantro leaves, and garlic cloves in a blender or food processor and blend first with the vinegar, then finish blending while adding the oil. Use over steak.

● ●

BONE BROTH

This recipe and accompanying notes courtesy of Adam Cole, LA-based chef and butcher.

When I told Adam that I was doing the ketogenic diet and needed some good-quality broth to go along with my diet of mainly fat, he immediately offered to make me some beef bone marrow broth. Mineral-rich, carbohydrate-free, fatty beef broth is to the ketogenic dieter what brown rice is to the vegetarian.

This broth bears no resemblance to the stuff you buy in a can or box at the grocery store. It's warming and delicious, and just the right thing on a day when you're feeling a little sluggish. Adam was nice enough to draw up the recipe with instructions that even a non-butcher (like me) could follow.

> 5 pounds beef bones (knuckle or vertebrae; you can get these at a butcher)
>
> vegetable oil, to coat
>
> 1 whole beef marrow bone (approximately 1 pound), cut lengthwise to expose marrow
>
> ice
>
> filtered water
>
> TOOLS
>
> 1 large metal sheet tray (like a cookie sheet)
>
> tongs
>
> slow cooker (6 quarts or larger; you can use a regular stock pot if you don't have a slow cooker)
>
> fine-mesh strainer or cheese cloth

Preheat oven to 400°F. Place 5 pounds of beef bones on sheet tray and coat lightly in vegetable oil. Roast bones in oven to caramelize, flipping with tongs occasionally to brown evenly. This should take about 45 minutes.

When bones are a deep brown color, carefully remove sheet tray from oven and place next to slow cooker. Transfer the roasted bones to the slow cooker using tongs, leaving the excess fat from roasting on the sheet tray. (Allow the sheet tray to cool completely before cleaning to prevent getting burned by hot beef fat.)

Place the split marrow bone on top of the roasted bones. Add as much ice as you can without it overflowing. Then, add water to cover the bones. (This should come up to about ½ inch from the top of the slow cooker.)

Place lid on slow cooker and turn on to the highest setting. Simmer broth for 24 hours.

After 24 hours, remove bones from broth with tongs and discard. Strain broth through fine-mesh strainer or cheese cloth. Do not discard the fat from the broth—that is all of the rendered bone marrow!

Cool and refrigerate until needed.

Notes on Marrow Broth

- If you have the option, ask your butcher to cut the bones into 1-inch pieces (they fit into the slow cooker more easily and allow for more flavor and gelatin extraction).

- If your bones (especially the vertebrae) have a little meat left on them, good! That's more flavor.

- For a "white broth," omit the roasting of the bones and place directly into slow cooker.

- The marrow bone itself is not roasted, because you want all of the marrow to render into your broth, rather than onto your sheet tray.

- The purpose of the ice, if you are wondering, is all about flavor and gelatin extraction. Starting your broth with very cold water ensures that you will pull as much flavor and gelatin (which translates into richness and depth) out of your bones as possible. It may take several hours for your broth to come up to a simmer because of this, but that is okay!

- Not all slow cookers are created equal. You want your broth to cook at a very low simmer. If the highest setting on your slow cooker is boiling your broth, reduce the heat so it is just bubbling a little bit and not reducing as it cooks.

- You can make this recipe in a stock pot on your stove, but because of the long cooking time required, a slow cooker is the safest and most effective way to go.

- Your finished broth will naturally separate as it cools, with the fat from the marrow rising to the top. This is a great way to store your broth, as the fat creates an airtight barrier and preserves the broth underneath. Refrigerated broth with a solid fat cap will last for several weeks. You can also freeze broth and store for up to a year.

- If you wish to emulsify the marrow fat into your broth, add ⅛ teaspoon or a very small pinch of xanthan gum to warm broth and blend with a blender or hand mixer to incorporate. Xanthan gum comes in powder form and can be found at specialty food stores and health stores, or online. Remember, a very small amount goes a long way.

- To season marrow broth, I like to use sea salt and Bragg's Liquid Aminos (a non-GMO, soy-based protein seasoning that is a gluten-free alternative to soy sauce).

- You can easily substitute pork, lamb, or chicken bones to create different flavors of broth.

Desserts & Sweets

● ●

CHOCOLATE COCONUT CUSTARD ICE CREAM

This recipe is from Dominic D'Agostino, Assistant Professor at the University of South Florida. Dominic researches the therapeutic benefits of ketones on human metabolism, and is a long-term ketogenic dieter himself. (See page 259 for my interview with Dominic.)

  1 can Thai condensed coconut milk

  1–2 squares unsweetened dark baking chocolate, melted

  4–6 drops stevia

  pinch of cinnamon

Open the can of Thai condensed coconut milk. The water may be on the bottom and the cream on top, so mix it to a uniform consistency. Mix all the ingredients together until they're the consistency of chocolate mousse and place in the freezer for a couple of hours. Dominic says it tastes pretty close to ice cream, and he eats just a little bit every night (it's very filling!).

> *Tip: You can find the condensed coconut milk in the Thai cooking section of the grocery store. It has the consistency of coconut cream.*

● ●

AVOCADO CHOCOLATE MOUSSE

I know what you're thinking: "Avocado in my dessert? C'mon!" Trust me, you won't even know it's there. The avocado replaces the cream and eggs called for in a typical mousse recipe, and you end up with a creamy, delicious keto dessert that's high in monounsaturated fat and low in saturated fat. This may help balance your diet if you've been ignoring my advice (shame on you!) to eat fat from both animal and vegetable sources and have instead focused on foods high in saturated fat, such as bacon, eggs, and the like.

    2 ripe avocados

    ¼ cup unsweetened cocoa

    3 tablespoons xylitol

    2 tablespoons unsweetened almond milk

    1 tablespoon bourbon

    1 teaspoon vanilla extract

Place all ingredients in a food processor and blend until very smooth. Chill at least 2 hours in the refrigerator before serving.

CHOCO-COCONUT POPSICLE

Maybe you remember making orange juice or Coca-Cola ice cubes as a kid? This version is just as fun to make, but it's much healthier and is suitable for the ketogenic diet.

    1 can full-fat coconut milk

    1 teaspoon coconut oil

    1½ tablespoons unsweetened cacao powder

Place all ingredients in a blender and blend until smooth. Place mixture into an ice cube tray and freeze for up to 3 hours. Place mixture into an ice cube tray and insert toothpicks into each cube. Freeze for at least 3 hours.

CHIA CHOCOLATE MOUSSE

I discovered this recipe by mistake one day because I became distracted while making a smoothie and left the blender on much too long. When I returned, I had mousse!

⅔ cup unsweetened almond milk

3 big handfuls baby spinach leaves

2 tablespoons almond meal (or ground almonds)

1 tablespoon cacao powder

1 tablespoon chia seeds

1 teaspoon ground cinnamon

pinch of cayenne pepper

pinch of salt

drop of stevia (optional)

Put milk in the blender first, then add spinach and remaining ingredients. Turn the blender on and pause once or twice to scrape down the sides where spinach will be stuck. Once you get all the leaves into the mix, leave the blender on for 3 minutes or more while the chia seeds thicken the mixture. It will slowly become stiff, sort of like a mousse or soft ice cream. Stop the blender when the mixture reaches your desired consistency (the consistency of Greek yogurt is a good target). You will have to scrape it from the bottom with a spoon.

Tip: Freeze for 15–20 minutes if you want something more ice cream–like.

Recipe Resources

You'll never want for recipe ideas, as dozens of sites out there are devoted to recipes for the ketogenic or low-carb dieter. The following are a good place to start.

- The Charlie Foundation website has a number of strict keto recipes with a very high ratio of fat to protein and carbs. (www.charliefoundation.org/resources-tools/resources-2/find-recipes).

- The blog attached to the site Ketodietapp.com has hundreds of recipes, but you must find your way to the blog page to access them (http://ketodietapp.com/Blog).

- The site ruled.me also offers hundreds of recipes, a lot of them leaning toward the indulgent end of the spectrum—think "chocolate-covered bacon" (www.ruled.me/keto-recipes).

- The Ketogenic Diet Resource features recipes organized by type of dish (e.g., breakfast, dessert, sauces) (www.ketogenic-diet-resource.com/low-carb-recipes.html).

CHAPTER 14

Community, Tools, and Resources for the New Ketogenic Dieter

You will undoubtedly search the web for more information as you continue on your diet and weight-loss journey. When seeking guidance on diet and health (and, frankly, any subject important to you), it's a good idea to ask yourself how credible the source is and if the author's philosophy aligns with your own.

Finding Credible Information Sources

The websites of major institutions, such as goverment agencies, universities, and education or advocacy organizations, are good sources for factual information on diet and health, though they generally take a conventional viewpoint. Blogs, newsletters, and websites written by individuals tend to offer more progressive viewpoints, although the accuracy of information from these sources may vary. When seeking health information you might consider the following:

- The author's training. Is he/she a trained scientist, nutritionist, physician, etc.? Does the author have credentials that are widely accepted as denoting expertise in the field, (e.g., PhD, RD, MD), or a variety of letters after their name that are incomprehensible?

- The author's tone. Do articles seems to "rant and rave" about the dangers of every imaginable food in a manner that is zealot-like, or is the voice a mature one that presents factual information in a way that's engaging, yet not overwhelming (such as in a newspaper article)?

- The author's business. This is one where you must use your judgment. In general, a company selling products has a vested interest in convincing you, the potential customer, to buy the thing they're selling. Does that mean that the information provided is not to be trusted? Not at all. What it means is that information is probably carefully selected to present one side of a story, and you may need to go elsewhere to get the remainder of the picture.

- The author's use of statistics and citing of references. Does the person make grand and surprising claims (e.g., "Did you know that blueberries cure cancer?") without backing them up with statistics or citations to credible references? If they do use references, are they to websites with similar styles of writing rather than to professional literature (such as scientific research studies or government or university databases)?

- The author's institutional culture. If the author is writing from within a government agency or non-governmental organization (NGO), consider the mission and culture of that institution. An author from within such an organization will often have to communicate a message that is both factually accurate *and* in line with the overall beliefs and goals of the institution. In addition, large entities such as government agencies tend to take longer than the private sector and individuals to integrate new knowledge into their messages. For that reason, government reports may be very useful for certain types of large-scale, standard data (such as the nutrient content of foods grown in the US) and not so useful for information that relies on rapidly changing knowledge (such as diet recommendations).

- The author's philosophy. There are many types of diets out there that can lead to weight loss and optimal health. Not all diets work for all people. Every group or individual has an approach that they believe is best. It's smart to find one that fits your needs and sensibilities.

It's certainly not the case that a person must have a degree in biochemistry or metabolism to write capably about diet and nutrition, nor that any author of nutritional content who writes emphatically about the need to reduce harmful foods in the diet is not to be trusted. Nor is it true that any information coming from a for-profit (or government or non-profit) entity is automatically biased or irrelevant. There is a great deal of accurate and useful information out there, and there is a lot of junk. It's worth taking a critical look at the sources you find yourself reading and using your best judgment to decide if they are providing trustworthy information that is particularly useful to you.

Online Resources

The Atkins Foundation
www.atkins.com

The Atkins site has just about everything a ketogenic dieter needs to succeed, including food lists with net carb counts, meal planners, recipes, suggestions for eating out, as well as an app for tracking your carb intake and an online community forum where members swap strategies for success on the Atkins diet. Everything except the forum is accessible right away; (free) registration is required to access the forum. You can also send away for a complimentary starter kit that includes the Atkins carb counter, a small book that lists hundreds of foods and their net carb counts. And if you're looking for a mobile app, the Atkins app is probably the biggest and most accurate of those dedicated to the low-carb dieter.

The Charlie Foundation for Ketogenic Therapies
www.charliefoundation.org

The Charlie Foundation exists to provide education on and promote the use of ketogenic diets for treatment of pediatric epilepsy, neurologic disorders, and tumorous cancers. The site is a valuable resource for information on ketogenic diets, but its focus is not on weight loss. Among its most relevant resources are: a list of low-carb and carb-free products (including mostly non-food items, such as over-the-counter medications and body care products); a large ketogenic recipe section; a recommended reading list; and a keto support line that covers topics relevant to any ketogenic dieter.

Jimmy Moore's Livin La Vida Low-Carb

www.livinlavidalowcarb.com

Jimmy Moore, a devoted low-carb dieter who is famous for losing 180 lbs in one year through ketogenic dieting, has written a number of books and hosts a wildly successful podcast on the subject of low-carb dieting (see my interview with Jimmy on page 62). His site features interviews with countless experts in the field and other valuable resources, such as a list of low-carb-proficient doctors nationwide. Jimmy also hosts a weeklong low-carb cruise each year, where low-carb diet experts present their latest research. Presentations from past cruises are highly informative and will be very helpful to the starting ketogenic dieter. These are accessible on Vimeo through the cruise's website (www.lowcarbcruiseinfo.com/) and on YouTube by searching "low-carb cruise."

Keto Nutrition

www.ketonutrition.org

This site is run by Dominic D'Agositino (see my interview with Dominic on page 259), a researcher at the University of South Florida who is an expert on ketogenic metabolism. A collection of resources focused largely on the ketogenic diet as a strategy of metabolic control, the site includes videos and podcasts that provide an in-depth look at the physiology of ketosis, not only for weight loss, but also for treatment of cancer, neurological diseases, and other disorders. In addition, the site provides links to online marketplaces where you can purchase ketogenic foods and supplements that may be difficult to find on your own.

Diet Doctor: Low-Carb, High-Fat Guide for Beginners
www.dietdoctor.com/lchf

Swedish family physician Andreas Eenfeldt maintains this site with the goal to help people achieve good health through the natural methods of diet and exercise. The overall site includes news stories, research studies, and facts about diet and weight loss, but the real gem is the LCHF (Low-Carb, High-Fat) beginners' page that offers a quick and comprehensive overview of the low-carb, high-fat approach to weight loss. There is also a fantastic set of video interviews Dr. Eenfeldt has done with other low-carb experts.

The Ketogenic Diet Resource
www.ketogenic-diet-resource.com

This online resource guide is run by Ellen Davis, "a self-taught nutrition writer freely offering information about food and nutrition with the hope of helping others feel better and live longer." The focus of the site is on how the ketogenic diet works, why it's beneficial, and what foods to eat while you're on it. It's chock-full of keto-friendly meal plans, recipes, and book recommendations. Sign up for Ellen's biweekly newsletter to get tips for the ketogenic dieter, success stories, products reviews, and other useful information.

KetoDiet: Real Food and Healthy Living Blog and App
http://ketodietapp.com

This site is maintained by low-carb enthusiast Martina Slajerova, who follows a ketogenic diet to manage an autoimmune condition. Martina is passionate about the value of ketogenic diets for weight maintenance and improved health. The site offers a variety of easy-to-use guides and a fantastic recipe section organized by type of dish (e.g., breakfast, dessert), amount of net carbs (e.g., 0–5 g, 5–10 g), and absence of problem ingredients (e.g., dairy-free, nut-free). Martina posts frequent updates of her experiments with keto cooking, as well as relevant news and nutrition information for the ketogenic dieter. Access to the blog is free, and the KetoDietApp is a new tool with recipes and tips available on both iPhone and iPad for $1.99.

Ruled.me
www.ruled.me

This site is run by Craig Clarke, an enthusiastic young man whose interest in the ketogenic diet helped him lose 100 lbs. The site offers a seemingly endless set of tips and recipes, as well as a handful of practical guides such as the Intermittent Fasting Guide and a 30-Day In-Depth Ketogenic Meal Plan. Craig has written two photo-filled keto cookbooks available for purchase on the site. A keto-dieter forum is in the works, and in the meantime you can join their Facebook group, which has over 10,000 members.

Paleo Magazine
http://paleomagonline.com

Paleo Magazine is probably the closest thing to a traditional media source targeting the ketogenic dieter. While not devoted to ketogenic diets per se, each issue provides a wealth of practical information useful to the high-fat, low-carb dieter, including shopping lists, recipes (many paleo recipes, with the exception of desserts, are keto-friendly), Q&As with health experts, reviews on new food products, and more. The magazine is distributed in digital and print versions six times a year and requires a subscription, but a monthly mini mag called the *Paleo Insider*, a podcast-style Paleo Radio, and tons of resources on the magazine's main website are all accessible for free.

Community

If you're looking to engage in a conversation with like-minded individuals, check out these sites to learn where you can fit in to the thriving low-carb community.

Active Low-Carbers Forum
http://forum.lowcarber.org

This is an online community of over 150,000 members who have lost over 2 million lbs by following a low-carb eating plan. The site is a support network for people on the Atkins, Protein Power, paleo, and similar diets that minimize sugar and starch. Members share their real-life experiences with low-carb dieting through conversation threads on various topics (e.g., tips for improving weight loss, details about carb amounts in different foods, the effects of caffeine or salt, success stories, recipes, what to do if you're not losing weight, etc.). These different perspectives can be a valuable tool in your ongoing learning, and can help you maintain and enjoy your low-carb lifestyle over the long term.

Reddit Keto Forums

Main site for keto dieters: www.reddit.com/r/keto

Keto recipes: www.reddit.com/r/ketorecipes

Female keto dieters: www.reddit.com/r/xxketo

There are multiple forums for keto dieters on Reddit: over 100,000 members use the main keto dieting site, over 37,000 contribute to the recipe site, and the women's specific site has over 12,000 members. The discussion threads cover everything from tips for getting started to product recommendations to suggestions for getting support from family members.

Mark's Daily Apple Forum

www.marksdailyapple.com

Over 180,000 members discuss paleo/primal living and dieting on this forum attached to the popular website, *Mark's Daily Apple*. The site is run by Mark Sisson (see my interview with Mark on page 267), a former endurance athlete and successful author, speaker, and leader in the primal living community. The site's mission is to inspire others to be happy, healthy, and fit—largely by increasing physical activity and reducing or eliminating sugar and grains from one's diet. Although this site is not dedicated to ketogenic diets per se, it is undeniably a rich resource for high-fat, low-carb dieters to share experiences and ask questions of one another to sustain the very-low-carb lifestyle over the long term.

Reference Sites for Nutrients in Foods

Finding accurate information about the nutrient and carb content of foods is essential to a successful ketogenic diet. You will inevitably face some challenges in your effort to find high-fat, wholesome foods in our largely processed-food environment. For nutrient information, tips on finding good foods, and to learn more about harmful food additives that may cause hormone disruption, weight gain, and otherwise threaten one's health, visit the following sites:

USDA National Nutrient Database for Standard Reference

http://ndb.nal.usda.gov/ndb/foods

The USDA is widely considered the most accurate source for nutrient content of whole foods, such as vegetables and meats. It provides calorie, macronutrient, and micronutrient content and gives the proportion of different fat types found in most foods. Foods are conveniently listed in various forms (e.g., raw, baked, boiled) in a variety of household measures (e.g., 1 tbsp, 1 cup, 3 oz). On the downside, the database is clunky and provides minimal data on packaged and restaurant items. It is best used for generic foods (e.g., 1 cup of broccoli). When researching packaged foods, it's essential to check the label on the actual product or visit the company website.

Environmental Working Group

www.ewg.org

The Environmental Working Group (EWG) researches and advocates on food safety and health issues. They publish a number of very useful consumer guides to help shoppers avoid genetically modified foods, pesticide residues in produce, and other potentially harmful food contaminants.

Center for Science in the Public Interest
www.cspinet.org

The Center for Science in the Public Interest (CSPI) is a research, education, and advocacy group that keeps track of the latest science on the health impacts of food additives (like alternative sweeteners), educates the public on nutrition trends (like the healthfulness of coconut oil), and announces changes to FDA regulations (such as food labeling laws), among other things. Their monthly Nutrition Action Newsletter covers timely topics in nutrition and health.

Books

Keto-Clarity: Your Definitive Guide to the Benefits of a Low-Carb, High-Fat Diet (2014)
by Jimmy Moore and Eric C. Westman, MD

Jimmy Moore has dedicated himself to sharing the benefits of ketogenic dieting with the world. In addition to his uber-popular website and podcast (see page 294 for more information), Jimmy's books *Cholesterol Clarity* (2013), and *21 Life Lessons from Livin' La Vida Low-Carb: How the Healthy Low-Carb Lifestyle Changed Everything I Thought I Knew* (2009), are foundational reading for the ketogenic dieter. His latest book, written with ketogenic diet expert Dr. Eric Westman, is an A–Z guide on ketogenic dieting and health.

The Art and Science of Low Carbohydrate Living
(2011) and The Art and Science of Low Carbohydrate Performance (2012)
by Jeff Volek and Stephen Phinney

Jeff Volek is Assistant Professor in the Department of Kinesiology at the University of Connecticut, and, along with Dr. Phinney, is a well-known researcher and expert in low-carb metabolism. The two study the physiologic effects of ketogenic diets on weight, health, and athletic performance, and their research is widely published in professional literature. Their books provide an in-depth and very scientific look at the metabolic effects of low-carb and ketogenic dieting.

New Atkins for a New You: The Ultimate Diet for Shedding Weight and Feeling Great (2010)
by Eric C. Westman, MD, Stephen D. Phinney, MD, and Jeff S. Volek, PhD

This is an updated and simplified guide to the popular Atkins diet. Dr. Westman (mentioned above) is the director of the Lifestyle Medicine Clinic at Duke University, and an expert in low-carb diets, diabetes, obesity, and insulin resistance. Drs. Phinney and Volek (mentioned above) are experts in low-carb metabolism and authors of multiple books on the subject.

Why We Get Fat: And What to Do About It (2010)
by Gary Taubes

Mr. Taubes is a courageous and renowned science journalist who has questioned conventional theories of weight gain for over a decade. Arguably as much of an expert on human metabolism as any practicing scientist, Mr. Taubes also has a knack for explaining difficult science concepts in understandable terms. This, his most recent book, explains which foods and behaviors contribute to weight gain and how we can reverse the problem.

The Stubborn Fat Fix: Eat Right to Lose Weight and Cure Metabolic Burnout without Hunger or Exercise (2009)
by Keith Berkowitz, MD, and Valerie Berkowitz, MS, RD

The book helps readers identify and correct metabolic imbalances to achieve weight loss and overall improved health. The authors worked with the pioneering ketogenic diet physician Dr. Robert Atkins at the Atkins Center for Complementary Medicine. They currently run the Center for Balanced Health in New York City, where they frequently use ketogenic or low-carb diets to help patients lose weight and reverse chronic disease.

Good Calories, Bad Calories: Fats, Carbs, and the Controversial Science of Diet and Health (2008)
by Gary Taubes

Taubes argues that refined carbohydrates like flour and sugar, rather than fat, are largely responsible for the rise in obesity and diabetes, and that the key to health lies in the types rather than amounts of calories we eat.

Journal Sources on Fat and Heart Health

Hu, T., Mills, K. T., Yao, L., Demanelis, K., Eloustaz, M., Yancy, W. S., Jr., Kelly, T. N., He, J., Bazzano, L. A. (October 2012). "Effects of low-carbohydrate diets versus low-fat diets on metabolic risk factors: A meta-analysis of randomized controlled clinical trials." *American Journal of Epidemiology.* 1(176) Supplement 7:S44–54.

Lawrence, G. D. (May 2013). "Dietary fats and health: Dietary recommendations in the context of scientific evidence." *Advances in Nutrition*. 4(3):294–302.

Malhotra, Aseem. (2013). "Saturated fat is not the major issue." *BMJ*. 347:f6340

Musunuru, Kiran. (October 2010). "Atherogenic dyslipidemia: Cardiovascular risk and dietary intervention." *Lipids*. 45(10):907–14.

Santos, F. L., Esteves, S. S., da Costa Pereira, A., Yancy, W. S., Jr., and Nunes, J. P. L. (2012). "Systematic review and meta-analysis of clinical trials of the effects of low carbohydrate diets on cardiovascular risk factors." *Obesity Reviews*. 13:1048–1066.

Siri-Tarino, P. W., Sun, Q., Hu, F. B., Krauss, R. M. (March 2010). "Meta-analysis of prospective cohort studies evaluating the association of saturated fat with cardiovascular disease." *American Journal of Clinical Nutrition*. 91(3):535–46.

Volek, J. S., Phinney, S. D., Forsythe, C. E., Quann, E. E., Wood, R. J., Puglisi, M. J., Kraemer, W. J., Bibus, D. M., Fernandez, M. L., Feinman, R. D. (April 2009). "Carbohydrate restriction has a more favorable impact on the metabolic syndrome than a low fat diet." *Lipids*. 44(4):297–309.

Yancy, W. S., Jr., Olsen, M. K., Guyton, J. R., Bakst, R. P., Westman, E. C. (May 18, 2004). "A low-carbohydrate, ketogenic diet versus a low-fat diet to treat obesity and hyperlipidemia: A randomized, controlled trial." *Annals of Internal Medicine*. 140(10):769–77.

Index

Insulin, 39–40, 75, 84, 155, 235–36; and fat metabolism, 82–83
Insulin resistance, 39–40, 79
Insulin resistance syndrome. *See* Metabolic syndrome
Italian restaurants, and low-carb diet, 225–26
Italian Spicy Sausage and Broccoli Rabe (recipe), 273–74

Jams/jellies, avoidance 169
Japanese restaurants, and low-carb diet, 226–28
Jimmy Moore's Livin La Vida Low-Carb (website), 294
Journal resources, 302–303

Kale chips, 191
Kelp noodles, 190
Keto Nutrition (website), 294
Keto-Clarity, 300
Ketoacidosis, 136–37
KetoDiet: Real Food and Healthy Living Blog and App, 289, 295–96
Ketogenic diet, 10–23; author's experiences, 1–9, 116–17, 213, 216–17; duration, 124–25; and eating out, 36, 106, 207–33; foods allowed, 13, 26–29, 30, 141–76, 194–206; foods to avoid, 13, 29–30, 168–76, 197; meal planning, 192–206; pantry preparation, 177–92, 243; quick-start guide, 24–37; recipes, 183, 184, 247, 271–89; resources, 245, 289, 290–303; tips, 234–48; transition period, 112–40
The Ketogenic Diet Resource (website), 289, 295
Ketogenic range, 65–66
Ketone urine strips, 35, 124, 139–40
Ketones, 35, 85; and cancer, 255–58; chemistry, 89; and energy, 76
Ketosis, 11–12, 17, 25, 35, 59, 65–66, 85–90; and carbohydrates, 30; excessive, 139–40; failure to enter, 134–35; and fats, 26; measuring, 124; and protein, 28; stopping, 66; vs. ketoacidosis, 136–37
"Ketosis," stigma, 63
"Ketostix." *See* Ketone urine strips
Kidneys, and ketosis, 31
Kilocalories, 74
Kitchen Sink Salad (recipe), 276–77

Acknowledgments

I am grateful to the courageous and forward-thinking individuals whose work helped me to keep an open and critical mind while I researched the ketogenic diet. Mr. Gary Taubes' persuasive and accessible writing on the history of the fat controversy in this country was, for me, a gateway to consideration of "the alternate hypothesis." I also thank Jimmy Moore, who shared his personal story so sincerely and honored me by writing the foreword to this book; Valerie Berkowitz, who helped me translate science into practice; Beth Zupec-Kania and Dominic D'Agostino, who were so generous with their time and expertise; and Dr. Thomas Seyfried, who graciously answered my elementary questions about the metabolism of cancer. I realized through these conversations that I was dealing with a community of thoughtful, intelligent professionals who, despite going against conventional wisdom, were making important and positive contributions to our understanding of diet and health.

I thank my dear friends Patricia Llanos, Naomi Hudson-Knapp, and Samantha Pitman for reading my writing; Lauren Swann for allowing me to guide her through the ketogenic diet; my partner, Cedar, for cooking me delicious fatty food and putting up with my almond addiction; and my good colleague Maggie Moon, who helped turn me into a science writer.

Finally, I thank the many individuals I have counseled in recent years. Your personal journeys to health have taught me more about change than I ever could have hoped to teach you. Thank you.

About the Author

Kristen Mancinelli, MS, RDN, is a public health nutritionist who writes about science and health to make seemingly obscure information useful to everyone. She has expertise in health behavior change, food and nutrition policy, and environmental nutrition. She received her bachelor of arts in chemistry from NYU and a master of science in nutrition and public health from Columbia University. Currently in Los Angeles, she counsels individuals in weight loss and prevention and management of chronic disease at UCLA. Learn more at www.kristenmancinelli.com.